Circadian Rhythm Disorders

Editor

PHYLLIS C. ZEE

NEUROLOGIC CLINICS

www.neurologic.theclinics.com

Consulting Editor
RANDOLPH W. EVANS

August 2019 • Volume 37 • Number 3

ELSEVIER

1600 John F. Kennedy Boulevard • Suite 1800 • Philadelphia, Pennsylvania, 19103-2899

http://www.theclinics.com

NEUROLOGIC CLINICS Volume 37, Number 3
August 2019 ISSN 0733-8619, ISBN-13: 978-0-323-68226-8

Editor: Stacy Eastman
Developmental Editor: Donald Mumford

Neurologic Clinics (ISSN 0733-8619) is published quarterly by Elsevier Inc., 360 Park Avenue South, New York, NY 10010–1710. Months of issue are February, May, August, and November. Periodicals postage paid at New York, NY, and additional mailing offices. Subscription prices are $323.00 per year for US individuals, $663.00 per year for US institutions, $100.00 per year for US students, $408.00 per year for Canadian individuals, $803.00 per year for Canadian institutions, $427.00 per year for international individuals, $803.00 per year for international institutions, and $210.00 for Canadian and foreign students/residents. To receive student/resident rate, orders must be accompanied by name of affiliated institution, date of term, and the *signature* of program/residency coordinator on institution letterhead. Orders will be billed at individual rate until proof of status is received. Foreign air speed delivery is included in all *Clinics* subscription prices. All prices are subject to change without notice. **POSTMASTER:** Send address changes to *Neurologic Clinics*, Elsevier Health Sciences Division, Subscription Customer Service, 3251 Riverport Lane, Maryland Heights, MO 63043. **Customer Service: Telephone: 1-800-654-2452 (U.S. and Canada); 314-447-8871 (outside U.S. and Canada). Fax: 314-447-8029. E-mail: journalscustomerservice-usa@elsevier.com (for print support); journalsonlinesupport-usa@elsevier.com (for online support).**

Reprints. For copies of 100 or more of articles in this publication, please contact the Commercial Reprints Department, Elsevier Inc., 360 Park Avenue South, New York, New York, 10010-1710; Tel.: +1-212-633-3874; Fax: +1-212-633-3820, and E-mail: reprints@elsevier.com.

Neurologic Clinics is also published in Spanish by Nueva Editorial Interamericana S.A., Mexico City, Mexico.

Neurologic Clinics is covered in *Current Contents/Clinical Medicine, MEDLINE/PubMed (Index Medicus), EMBASE/Excerpta Medica,* and *PsycINFO,* and *ISI/BIOMED.*

Contributors

CONSULTING EDITOR

RANDOLPH W. EVANS, MD
Clinical Professor, Department of Neurology, Baylor College of Medicine, Houston, Texas

EDITOR

PHYLLIS C. ZEE, MD, PhD
Benjamin and Virginia T. Boshes Professor in Neurology, Chief, Division of Sleep Medicine in the Department of Neurology, Director, Center for Circadian and Sleep Medicine, Northwestern University Feinberg School of Medicine, Chicago, Illinois

AUTHORS

SABRA M. ABBOTT, MD, PhD
Assistant Professor, Department of Neurology, Northwestern University Feinberg School of Medicine, Chicago, Illinois

PHILIP CHENG, PhD
Assistant Scientist, Sleep Disorders and Research Center, Henry Ford Health System, Detroit, Michigan

ELIZABETH CULNAN, PhD
Postdoctoral Fellow, Department of Psychiatry and Behavioral Sciences, Rush University Medical Center, Chicago, Illinois

CHRISTOPHER DRAKE, PhD
Director of Sleep Research, Sleep Disorders and Research Center, Henry Ford Health System, Detroit, Michigan

JOHN B. HOGENESCH, PhD
Divisions of Human Genetics and Immunobiology, Department of Pediatrics, Center for Chronobiology, Cincinnati Children's Hospital Medical Center, Cincinnati, Ohio

PENG JIANG, PhD
Research Assistant Professor, Center for Sleep and Circadian Biology, Department of Neurobiology, Weinberg College of Arts and Sciences, Northwestern University, Evanston, Illinois

ELIZABETH B. KLERMAN, MD, PhD
Associate Professor, Division of Sleep and Circadian Disorders, Department of Medicine, Brigham and Women's Hospital, Boston, Massachusetts

LINDSAY M. McCULLOUGH, MD
Sleep Medicine Fellow, Department of Medicine, Rush University Medical Center, Chicago, Illinois

TEMITAYO OYEGBILE, MD, PhD
Assistant Professor of Neurology, Georgetown University, Medical Director, MedStar St. Mary's Sleep Lab, Georgetown University Medical Center, Washington, DC

MELANIE POGACH, MD, MMSc
Department of Internal Medicine, Division of Pulmonary, Critical Care and Sleep, Beth Israel Deaconess Medical Center, Boston, Massachusetts

KATHRYN J. REID, PhD
Research Professor, Department of Neurology, Center for Circadian and Sleep Medicine, Northwestern University Feinberg School of Medicine, Chicago, Illinois

MARC D. RUBEN, PhD
Divisions of Human Genetics and Immunobiology, Department of Pediatrics, Center for Chronobiology, Cincinnati Children's Hospital Medical Center, Cincinnati, Ohio

WILLIAM J. SCHWARTZ, MD
Professor, Department of Neurology, Dell Medical School, Department of Integrative Biology, College of Natural Sciences, The University of Texas at Austin, Austin, Texas

KAZUHIRO SHIMOMURA, DVM, PhD
Research Assistant Professor, Center for Sleep and Circadian Biology, Department of Neurology, Northwestern University Feinberg School of Medicine, Chicago, Illinois

DAVID F. SMITH, MD, PhD
Divisions of Pediatric Otolaryngology and Pulmonary and Sleep Medicine, Cincinnati Children's Hospital Medical Center, Department of Otolaryngology–Head and Neck Surgery, University of Cincinnati School of Medicine, Cincinnati, Ohio

ROBERT JOSEPH THOMAS, MD, MMSc
Department of Internal Medicine, Division of Pulmonary, Critical Care and Sleep, Beth Israel Deaconess Medical Center, Boston, Massachusetts

ALEKSANDAR VIDENOVIC, MD, MSc
Associate Professor of Neurology, Harvard Medical School, Chief, Division of Sleep Medicine, Massachusetts General Hospital, Boston, Massachusetts

MARTHA HOTZ VITATERNA, PhD
Research Professor, Center for Sleep and Circadian Biology, Department of Neurobiology, Weinberg College of Arts and Sciences, Northwestern University, Evanston, Illinois

JAMES K. WYATT, PhD, FAASM
Associate Professor and Director, Section of Sleep Disorders and Sleep-Wake Research, Department of Psychiatry and Behavioral Sciences, Rush University Medical Center, Chicago, Illinois

PHYLLIS C. ZEE, MD, PhD
Benjamin and Virginia T. Boshes Professor in Neurology, Chief, Division of Sleep Medicine in the Department of Neurology, Director, Center for Circadian and Sleep Medicine, Northwestern University Feinberg School of Medicine, Chicago, Illinois

Contents

Endogenous central and peripheral circadian oscillators are key to organizing multiple aspects of mammalian physiology; this clock tracks the day-night cycle and governs behavioral and physiologic rhythmicity. Flexibility in the timing and duration of sleep and wakefulness, critical to the survival of species, is the result of a complex, dynamic interaction between 2 regulatory processes: the clock and a homeostatic drive that increases with wake duration and decreases during sleep. When circadian rhythmicity and sleep homeostasis are misaligned—as in shifted schedules, time zone transitions, aging, or disease—sleep, metabolic, and other disorders may ensue.

In mammals, genetic influences of circadian rhythms occur at many levels. A set of core "clock genes" have been identified that form a feedback loop of gene transcription and translation. The core genetic clockwork generates circadian rhythms in cells throughout the body. Polymorphisms in both core clock genes and interacting genes contribute to individual differences in the expression and properties of circadian rhythms. The circadian clock profoundly influences the patterns of gene expression and cellular functions, providing a mechanistic basis for the impact of the genetic circadian system on normal physiological processes as well as the development of diseases.

Circadian rhythms are observed in most physiologic functions across a variety of species and are controlled by a master pacemaker in the brain called the suprachiasmatic nucleus. The complex nature of the circadian system and the impact of circadian disruption on sleep, health, and well-being support the need to assess internal circadian timing in the clinical setting. The ability to assess circadian rhythms and the degree of circadian disruption can help in categorizing subtypes or even new circadian rhythm disorders and aid in the clinical management of the these disorders.

This article reviews delayed and advanced sleep-wake phase disorders. Diagnostic procedures include a clinical interview to verify the misalignment of the major nocturnal sleep episode relative to the desired and social-normed timing of sleep, a 3-month or greater duration of the sleep-wake disturbance, and at least a week of sleep diary data consistent with the sleep timing complaint. Treatment options include gradual, daily shifting of the sleep schedule (chronotherapy); shifting circadian phase with properly timed light exposure (phototherapy); or melatonin administration. Future directions are discussed to conclude the article.

Non–24-hour sleep-wake rhythm disorder is a circadian rhythm sleep-wake disorder characterized by an inability to entrain to the 24-hour environment. Patients present with complaints of insomnia or hypersomnia, with progressive daily shifts of sleep-wake activity on actigraphy or sleep logs. Although first recognized in blind individuals without light perception, it also can be seen in individuals with intact vision. Treatment focuses on timed melatonin in blind individuals, whereas it is more complex in sighted individuals, using multiple time cues, such as light, melatonin, social interactions, feeding, and activity.

This article focuses on irregular sleep-wake rhythm disorder (ISWRD) and its associations with several other comorbidities. Irregular sleep-wake rhythm disorder is a circadian disorder characterized by a lack of a clear sleep-wake pattern. The disorder has yet to be fully understood from pathophysiologic perspective. Treatments are available, but there is a need for development of novel interventions. The goal of this article is to focus on multiple aspects of ISWRD.

Shift work and its negative consequences are becoming more relevant as the economy becomes increasing globalized. For many individuals, shift work serves as a significant biological and psychosocial challenge leading to Shift Work Disorder (SWD). Beyond the symptoms of sleep and excessive sleepiness, the range of consequences for health and daily functioning in those with SWD are reviewed, along with evidence-based recommendations for clinical management, including comprehensive clinical assessments and intervention strategies that target multiple domains through pharmacologic and nonpharmacologic methods. A review of important recent scientific and technological developments for assessment and intervention is also provided.

The complex interplay of the sleep and circadian systems, which are substantially differentially regulated, provides for plasticity that is expressed in health and disease. The classic circadian rhythm disorders are readily recognizable, but atypical forms can be identified by actigraphy and melatonin profilometry. Although the dim-light melatonin onset test maps the start of the biological night, 24-hour mapping can define the limits of the biological night, whereas other forms of strategic testing can identify conditions such as iatrogenic hypermelatoninemia. Routine testing in clinical practice can expand the range of identifiable circadian rhythm disorders.

Circadian rhythms are present in nearly all organisms studied, and are present throughout the human body. The proper coordination of these rhythms, both within the body, and with respect to the environment appears to be important for overall health. This article reviews the available data looking at the association between circadian dysregulation and cardiometabolic, neurologic, and neurodegenerative disease risk. In addition we discuss the limited but growing evidence supporting the use of circadian-based interventions to improve overall health.

Fundamental aspects of neurobiology are time-of-day regulated. Therefore, it is not surprising that neurodegenerative and psychiatric diseases are accompanied by sleep and circadian rhythm disruption. Although the direction of causation remains unclear, abnormal sleep-wake patterns often occur early in disease, exacerbate progression, and are a common primary complaint from patients. Circadian medicine incorporates knowledge of 24-hour biological rhythms to improve treatment. This article highlights how research and technologic advances in circadian biology might translate to improved patient care.

NEUROLOGIC CLINICS

RELATED SERIES

Neuroimaging Clinics
Psychiatric Clinics
Child and Adolescent Psychiatric Clinics

THE CLINICS ARE AVAILABLE ONLINE!
Access your subscription at:
www.theclinics.com

Preface

A Perfect Time for Circadian Medicine

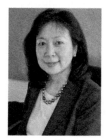

Phyllis C. Zee, MD, PhD
Editor

This issue of *Neurologic Clinics* is devoted to the important emerging field of circadian medicine and its implications to the practice of neurology, and medicine as a whole. This issue comes on the heels of the 2017 Nobel Prize in Physiology or Medicine, which recognized the seminal discovery of the genetic mechanisms that generate circadian rhythms and the overarching impact of biological timing to the practice of medicine. Since the mid 1990s, and in particular during the past decade, discoveries demonstrated the ubiquity of these molecular circadian clocks in nearly all tissues of the nervous system and throughout the body. The evidence that circadian genes not only regulate timing but also are integrally involved in metabolic, inflammatory, and cellular repair processes, and that more than a third of protein-encoding genes exhibiting circadian rhythmicity underscores the importance of the time domain in medicine. Just during the past decade, evidence from basic, clinical, and epidemiologic studies indicates that circadian rhythm and sleep disturbances are not just mere consequences of neurologic disease but also contribute to the expression of common neurologic disorders and the pathogenesis of neurodegenerative disorders.

In addition to innate circadian disturbances, technological advances in modern societies have increased the demand "working" against our circadian biology, resulting in circadian rhythm disorders (CRD). Some CRDs are due to misalignment between the timing of the endogenous circadian rhythm and the external environment, while others result from dysfunction of the brain's master circadian clock, its input and output pathways, or genetic mutations of clock genes that alter downstream physiology and behavior. Given the high prevalence of circadian and sleep disturbances among patients with neurologic disorders, several of the articles in this issue emphasize that CRDs should be considered in the differential diagnosis of all patients with symptoms of insomnia or excessive daytime sleepiness. Treatment approaches that target

https://doi.org/10.1016/j.ncl.2019.05.003
0733-8619/19/© 2019 Published by Elsevier Inc.

circadian amplitude and synchronization can improve sleep quality, but also neurologic and other health outcomes.

I am most grateful to my colleagues for their enthusiastic and valuable contributions to this issue. They have succeeded in providing up-to-date reviews on the current knowledge of circadian science, diagnosis, and treatment of common and challenging CRDs and a view into the future of circadian diagnostics and therapeutics in medicine. I would like to thank the senior developmental editor, Donald Mumford, for his patience and advice throughout the preparation of this issue and to acknowledge the *Neurologic Clinics* editors for their vision to dedicate an entire issue to circadian rhythm disorders.

Phyllis C. Zee, MD, PhD
Division of Sleep Medicine
Department of Neurology
Center for Circadian and Sleep Medicine
Northwestern University
Feinberg School of Medicine
710 North Lake Shore Drive
Suite 520
Chicago, IL 60611, USA

E-mail address:
p-zee@northwestern.edu

Circadian Neurobiology and the Physiologic Regulation of Sleep and Wakefulness

William J. Schwartz, MD[a,b,*], Elizabeth B. Klerman, MD, PhD[c]

KEYWORDS

• Circadian rhythms • Suprachiasmatic nucleus • Sleep • Homeostasis • Physiology

KEY POINTS

• Precise, robust, and flexible circadian rhythmicity is the product of a network of tissue and organ clocks, including a master clock in the suprachiasmatic nucleus of the hypothalamus.

• The timing, duration, and content of sleep are regulated by nonlinear interactions between circadian and sleep homeostatic processes and the environmental and behavioral variables that affect them.

• Changes in the time course, strength, or alignment of circadian and homeostatic drives, either environmentally or pathologically, can begin to account for disordered sleep rhythms and suggest rational therapeutic approaches.

INTRODUCTION

The Earth's 24-hour axial rotation has forced most organisms to evolve and adapt to a dramatic recurring cycle of day and night. Endogenous circadian timekeeping systems are one of evolution's responses to this challenge; these timekeeping systems allow living things to recognize local environmental time and to measure time's passage. The result is an ability to anticipate periodic daily events, orchestrate internal temporal programs of behavioral activities and metabolic (and other physiologic)

Disclosure Statement: This article is funded by NIH Grant numbers: P01-AG009975; R21-HD086392; K24-HL105664; R01-GM105018; R01-HL128538.
Funded by: NIHHYB Grant number(s): NIA P01-AG009975; NICHD R21-HD086392; NIH K24-HL105664; R01-GM-105018; R01-HL128538 NIHMS-ID: 1524361
[a] Department of Neurology, Dell Medical School, The University of Texas at Austin, Health Discovery Building 5.702, 1601 Trinity Street Building B, Austin, TX 78712, USA; [b] Department of Integrative Biology, College of Natural Sciences, The University of Texas at Austin, Austin, TX, USA; [c] Division of Sleep and Circadian Disorders, Department of Medicine, Brigham and Women's Hospital, 221 Longwood Avenue, Boston, MA 02115, USA
* Corresponding authors. Department of Neurology, Dell Medical School, The University of Texas at Austin, Health Discovery Building 5.702, 1601 Trinity Street Building B, Austin, TX 78712.
E-mail addresses: william.schwartz@austin.utexas.edu (W.J.S.); ebklerman@hms.harvard.edu (E.B.K.)

functions, and flexibly set the order and scheduling of such activities and functions to (presumably) optimize fitness in the natural world.[1,2] This system is vital to adjusting the timing and duration of bouts of rest and activity, eating, and other functions to the ecological niche. The system also lies at the core of various mechanisms for successful adaptation to the seasons[3,4]; it enables tracking the changing day length to activate winter strategies to conserve energy, change coloration to avoid detection by predators, time reproductive events, and/or escape by migrating thousands of miles away (using the sun as a time-compensated compass for navigating across the latitudes). The circadian clock is indeed a clock for all seasons.

THE FORMAL LANGUAGE OF CIRCADIAN CLOCKS AND RHYTHMS

Circadian rhythms are innate, persisting with an approximately 24-hour oscillation in organisms and across generations in constant environmental conditions (eg, the rhythms free-run in constant darkness), and are accurate and precise, even in the face of changing temperatures. Like all rhythmic phenomena, their properties can be described in mathematical terms, such as period, phase, and amplitude (**Fig. 1**).

Circadian rhythmicity represents the overt manifestation of an internal pacemaker that functions as a clock through the daily resetting of its approximately 24-hour oscillation by environmental 24-hour cues, thus adopting a stable phase relationship to the environment (ie, entrainment). Of the possible multitude of entraining cues (zeitgebers), light is the most powerful and the best studied. Photic phase response curves rigorously quantify the resetting responses of rhythms to light pulses presented across the circadian cycle, revealing how the interaction of an endogenous oscillation with a rhythm of light responsiveness can lead to precise and accurate entrainment to the natural light:dark (day:night) cycle and shift it to a new phase (eg, after travel across time zones). For entrainment, the clock is reset to match its intrinsic period to 24 hours; light administered just before dawn advances its rhythm, whereas exposure to an identical light stimulus (in duration, wavelength, and intensity) after dusk delays its rhythm. So, to entrain the clock of an animal with an endogenous free-running period longer than 24 hours (as is typical for humans), daily morning light acts to increase the clock's speed and advance its phase. Importantly, a stimulus also can affect the expression of a rhythm without entraining its underlying clock; such a mechanism has been termed, *masking*, because it bypasses or acts downstream of the clock and thus masks the clock's true state. For example, studies of the core body temperature (CBT) rhythm in humans (which is significantly influenced by the circadian clock) have revealed that masking factors, such as light at night, activity levels, postural changes, meal times, and sleep, may alter its value significantly[5]; therefore, determining the endogenous circadian rhythm in CBT requires specialized conditions in which these masking factors are minimized or spread evenly over 24 hours (discussed later).

Although historically the search for the clock focused on its self-sustained rhythmicity, it is the phase of entrainment (eg, the timing of sleep onset, temperature minimum, or locomotor activity peak in relation to the light:dark cycle) that matters for survival in the wild.[6] The clock's free-running period and phase of entrainment are systematically related to each other, such that faster clocks (shorter period length) tend to lead to earlier phase of entrainment; but entrainment phase also is affected by other factors, including the intensity of light and prior exposure to different day lengths. The entrainment phase is sometimes referred to as *chronotype*, or the temporal phenotype of an individual or a population (as in morning larks and night owls), and has provided a window for understanding how genetic determinants and ecological constraints (including those imposed by own urban living and societal mores) shape rhythmic behaviors.[7]

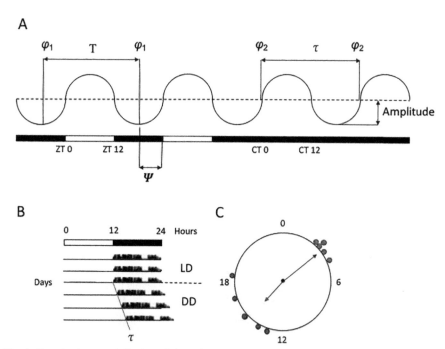

Fig. 1. Terminology and displays. (*A*) A schematic circadian rhythm, on the left, entrained to a 12-hour:12-hour light:dark cycle and, on the right, free-running under constant darkness. White bar, light; black bar, dark. Under entrainment, zeitgeber time (ZT) 0 represents the time of lights on (dawn) and ZT 12 the time of lights off (dusk); during free-running, circadian time (CT) 0 represents subjective dawn and CT 12 subjective dusk. T, period length of the zeitgeber; τ, period length of the free-running rhythm; φ, phase, a defined, stable cycle-to-cycle reference point within the cycle of the rhythm (eg, φ_1, the minimum value); Ψ, phase angle of entrainment, the time difference (phase relationship) between a defined phase of the rhythm and an external phase-reference (eg, zt 0). (*B*) A schematic circadian rhythm in actogram format. Data (eg, locomotor activity) are plotted horizontally from left to right over the course of 24-hour periods, with succeeding days stacked vertically from top to bottom. LD, light:dark cycle; DD, constant darkness. (*C*) A schematic circular plot of the phases of individual rhythms from 2 populations, from 0 to 24 hours (or sometimes graphed from 0° to 360°). The solid radial arrow represents the mean phase of each population and its length a measure of the scatter within each population. This format for plotting angular data illustrates that a mean of 15 for the red population is not a larger value than a mean of 3 for the blue population but rather a difference in their relative phases.

A NETWORK FOR INTERNAL TIME

Although daily rhythms—the opening and closing of leaves in concert with the alternation of day and night, for example—have been known since antiquity, the mechanistic understanding of daily and annual timing has blossomed over the past 50 years, now encompassing details at the molecular, cellular, tissue, organismal, and even societal levels. The basic oscillatory mechanism is intracellular, focused on a suite of clock genes that function within negative autoregulatory feedback loops, rhythmically repressing the transcription of their own mRNAs[8] (see Allada, this issue). Post-transcriptional and post-translational regulatory mechanisms, currently under active investigation by many researchers, also clearly contribute to fundamental rhythm properties. Clock transcription factors do not operate solely within the clock's feedback loops; they regulate the transcription of downstream clock-controlled genes in a wide array of the cell's metabolic and other pathways. This linkage begins to suggest how the motion of a molecular clock can be translated into a 24-hour program of biochemical events.

The identification of clock genes enabled the construction of transgenic mice bearing bioluminescent reporters (eg, using clock gene promoter elements to drive rhythmic transcription of the gene encoding the enzyme luciferase), contributing to the discovery that cells, tissues, and organs throughout the brain and body express circadian oscillators.[9] In mammals, the suprachiasmatic nucleus (SCN) of the anterior hypothalamus (discussed later) orchestrates this network for internal time, in which the multiplicity of peripheral clocks exhibit defined but permutable phase relationships to each other and the environmental light:dark cycle. This coordination is mediated by the interplay of several coupling factors that carry the SCN's output signals to subsidiary clocks—including rhythms of behavior (eg, rest and activity, feeding, and fasting), CBT, hormone levels (eg, cortisol, melatonin), and neural activity—in various combinations and strengths[10] (**Fig. 2**). This system can ensure homeostasis over time; as an example, the hepatic clock's proper timing of compensatory glycogenolysis and glucose export enables maintenance of plasma glucose levels through nighttime fasting.[11,12] By tuning coupling strengths and oscillator speeds, the network should be capable of adaptively realigning the relative phasing of its components under changing internal and external conditions. Such short-term circumstances might include food availability at an unexpected time as well as social interactions; note that during development, the phase of the hepatic clock in rat pups reverses around the time of weaning, corresponding to the switch from diurnal nursing to nocturnal feeding.[13] On the other hand, pathologic misalignment—between the environment and behavior, between behavior and the SCN, between the SCN and peripheral clocks, or between peripheral clocks—might be both a consequence and a cause of at least some of the symptoms of aging and disease (see Zee, this issue).

THE SUPRACHIASMATIC NUCLEUS AS A MAMMALIAN MASTER CLOCK

The SCN is a bilaterally paired hypothalamic nucleus straddling the midline, bordering the third ventricle above the optic chiasm.[14] Although present in diverse species, it has been studied most intensively in rodents. Its metabolic and neuronal spike activities exhibit circadian rhythms in vivo and in vitro; in vivo, there is a close congruence between the rhythm of electrical activity and the temporal profile of behavioral rest and activity, with feedback effects of locomotion and sleep shaping the waveform of SCN firing rate.[15,16] Behavioral, physiologic, and hormonal circadian rhythms depend on the integrity of the SCN; ablation of the nucleus results in circadian arrhythmicity without disrupting homeostatic mechanisms, whereas neural grafts of fetal SCN tissue re-establish behavioral rhythmicity in arrhythmic SCN-lesioned recipients, with the rhythms restored by the transplants exhibiting properties characteristic of the circadian pacemakers of the donors rather than those of the hosts.[17]

Photic entrainment of SCN rhythmicity relies on a monosynaptic retinal input that primarily codes for luminance, involves signaling by glutamate and pituitary adenylate cyclase-activating peptide, and reflects the activity of a class of melanopsin-expressing, intrinsically photoreceptive retinal ganglion cells (ipRGCs); other ipRGCs seem to subserve light-modulatory effects on aspects of sleep and mood.[18] SCN neural outputs are mostly intrahypothalamic but with close connections to key targets. Via the ventral subparaventricular zone, these include polysynaptic pathways to

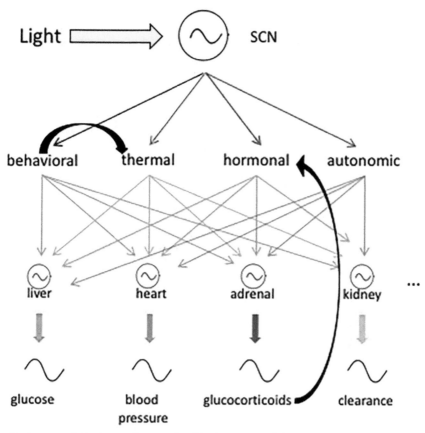

Fig. 2. A network for internal time. Simplified cartoon of the mammalian circadian time-keeping system, with the SCN entrained by the light:dark cycle and peripheral body clocks entrained by SCN output signals, including rhythmic behaviors, CBT, hormone levels, and nervous system activity; not shown are other clocks within the nervous system itself. These subsidiary clocks and rhythms also can respond to inputs downstream of the SCN (eg, a shifted cycle of food availability on the hepatic clock). Of possible feedbacks, 2 exemplary ones are illustrated (ie, locomotor activity itself affecting CBT; adrenal output itself acting as a coupling signal).

sleep-active and wake-active cell groups, suggesting a circadian influence on both behavioral states that is time dependent.[19,20] The phases of intrinsic SCN rhythms are similar in diurnally active and nocturnally active species, suggesting that the differing chronotypes of these species require inversion of SCN output signals or their reception.[21] Another important output is via the sympathetic system and its innervation of the pineal gland, which drives the nocturnal synthesis and secretion of melatonin. Both diurnal and nocturnal species display high melatonin levels during the night (dark phase), with its duration inversely related to the length of the day (light phase).[3,4] There also is evidence implicating SCN output via diffusible substances, for example, transforming growth factor α[22] and prokineticin 2.[23]

The circadian clock in the SCN is itself a complex coupled network of heterogeneous neuronal (and glial) oscillators.[24,25] Anatomic modules have been defined by neuro-transmitters and other biomarkers, with functional consequences following their specific genetic manipulation: a retino-recipient region (referred to as *core*) that includes neurons expressing vasoactive intestinal polypeptide and gastrin-releasing peptide and an arginine vasopressin neuronal shell and other identified cell groups that overlap these subdivisions (eg, expressing neuromedin S or D1 dopamine receptor). Somehow these anatomic units are dynamically coupled to yield emergent properties of the SCN clock that are critical to its function. Circuit-level mechanisms enable clock precision (generation of a stable ensemble period from sloppy cellular oscillations), robustness (persistence in the face of genetic perturbations), and plasticity (cellular-phase dispersion in response to changing day length). One such mechanism involves the interaction of SCN molecular and electrical activities. The intracellular molecular clock governs electrical activity through an array of ion channels that switch resting membrane potential from daytime depolarization to nighttime hyperpolarization and sustain the level of neuronal firing; in turn, electrical activity regulates calcium-dependent transcription and thus the phase and amplitude of the molecular clock. Under investigation are additional mechanisms (eg, state-dependent actions of vasoactive intestinal polypeptide and γ-aminobutyric acid, small-world network topology) to account for the complex spatiotemporal activity patterns exhibited by SCN tissue.

ON SLEEP AND WAKEFULNESS

The most obvious circadian-regulated output is sleep and wake timing. Sleep is a complex multisite and multifunction behavior. Overtly, it involves changes in consciousness, responsiveness, and posture. Within the organism, it causes changes in all physiologic systems. Unlike coma and anesthesia, sleep is unique in its ability to, without external pharmacologic manipulation, rapidly and reversibly change to a fully functioning wake state.[26] Considerable progress is being made in elucidating the neural circuitry underlying the regulation of sleep:wake states and their transitions.[27,28]

Sleep is required for normal physiology; death occurs if there is long-term sleep deprivation.[29] The multiple changes that occur during sleep are important for the entire body, not just for the brain. Surprisingly, the function of sleep is unknown. As Dr Alan Rechtschaffen famously said, "If sleep doesn't serve an absolutely vital function, it is the greatest mistake evolution ever made."[30] During the time animals sleep, they are not procreating, feeding, or defending themselves—3 important behaviors for sustaining the species. Therefore, the fact that sleep or sleep-like behavior has persisted in every animal species suggests that it is required for normal physiologic functioning. There are probably multiple functions of—or, more properly, functions that occur during—sleep, suggesting that sleep is the platform during which multiple physiologic processes occur. Sleep is not just required for feeling rested; metabolic, immunologic, cognitive, and other physiologic work occur during sleep. Each of these physiologic processes probably has its own time course of buildup and decay, so enough sleep for one function may be different than for another. Therefore, completing these functions would be expected to be part of the regulation of timing or duration of sleep. Even sleep is not uniform; it is composed of rapid eye movement (REM) sleep and non-REM (NREM) sleep, which are differentially regulated (discussed later). More studies are needed to determine the time course of buildup and decay of each of these processes, because the timing and duration of sleep would also be expected to be regulated to increase the chance of survival.

CIRCADIAN AND HOMEOSTATIC REGULATION OF SLEEP TIMING AND CONTENT

The two-process model[31] is the dominant framework for understanding the timing and content of sleep behavior at the level of the whole organism and specific brain areas.

The 2 processes are circadian rhythmicity (process C) and sleep homeostasis (process S). Sleep homeostasis increases during wake (and possibly REM sleep) and decreases during sleep (or possibly just NREM sleep). Accepted markers of sleep homeostasis across 1 or 2 sleep and wake episodes (eg, wake episodes lasting 4–60 hours and daytime and/or nighttime sleep episodes) are slow wave sleep (SWS) (N3 under current American Academy of Sleep Medicine criteria) or slow wave activity (SWA) (approximately 0.5–4.5 Hz during sleep and/or approximately 12.25–25.0 Hz[32] during wake in the electroencephalogram [EEG]); the putative biochemical agent is adenosine. All these markers have levels that increase with wake duration and decrease during sleep. Consistent with this is that caffeine, an adenosine receptor antagonist, decreases sleepiness. The buildup and decay of process S are modeled mathematically as saturating exponentials—consistent with data that lost sleep is not recovered minute-by-minute and, therefore, an intensity factor (eg, increased SWA) must be involved. For a longer time course of sleep homeostasis, as seen with chronic sleep restriction (ie, multiple nights with insufficient sleep), SWS and SWA are not appropriate markers and the time course of buildup and recovery is different than for sleep deprivation (ie, 1 continuous wake episode)[33]; a hypothesized biochemical change is in adenosine receptor concentrations.[34]

PROTOCOLS FOR SEPARATING CIRCADIAN AND SLEEP:WAKE INFLUENCES

A difficulty in determining the relative effect of circadian rhythmicity and sleep homeostatic factors is that circadian timing (phase) and sleep homeostatic buildup and decay covary: on a 24-hour schedule with sleep at night and wake during the day, both circadian phase and the length of time awake (during which sleep homeostasis increases) or asleep (during which sleep homeostasis decreases) advance at the same rate. For example, suppose circadian time 0 is set as 5:00 AM, wake time at 7:00 AM, and sleep onset time at 11:00 PM. Then wake time is at circadian time 2; 5 hours after wake time is circadian time 7; and sleep onset time (after 16 hours awake) is circadian time 18. It can never be learned what happens when circadian time is 18 but wake duration is 2 hours, such as might happen with someone working the night shift or experiencing jet lag. An additional difficulty in determining circadian phase or sleep:wake influence on a variable is that sleep and wake are associated with multiple other differences besides the sleep or wake state; these include differences in physical and mental activity levels, fasting/feeding, social interactions, lighting conditions, and posture. Therefore, sleep or wake per se may not be the only determining factor influencing the variable(s) of interest.

For these reasons, several types of protocols have been developed to separate the circadian and homeostatic influences on sleep:wake physiology. In two of these protocols, subjects are not allowed to choose their sleep and wake times, change lighting conditions (which usually are very dim to minimize alerting and phase-shifting effects of light), or know clock time. One protocol is the constant routine, in which the subjects remain awake for 40 hours or longer in constant posture and dim light conditions and eat multiple small meals; this enables study of wake at all circadian phases and especially at 2 different sleep homeostatic pressures (24 hours apart) for each circadian phase and under conditions in which masking (defined previously) is minimized or distributed equally across all circadian phases. This protocol, however, induces sleep deprivation; it, therefore, is of great use for studying hormones, performance, and cardiovascular, metabolic, immune, and other physiologic functions but of limited use for studying the independent effects of circadian rhythmicity and sleep homeostasis on sleep. The other protocol is a forced desynchrony protocol in which subjects live on non–24-hour days. Studies have been conducted with days as short as 90 minutes[35] and as long as 42.85 hours.[33] Within each of these days, there usually is a 2:1 wake:-sleep (and light:dark) ratio, although other ratios can be used if chronic sleep restriction is being studied.[36] Under such schedules, the circadian pacemaker cannot entrain to the wake:sleep or light:dark cycle, leading to desynchrony between circadian and sleep homeostatic processes. These forced desynchrony protocols create multiple evenly distributed combinations of length of time awake or asleep at each circadian phase, so that separate effects of circadian rhythmicity and sleep homeostasis can be studied. Such intensive inpatient studies have documented the findings (described later) about the relative circadian and homeostatic influences on sleep timing and duration.

A third protocol in which individuals sometimes exhibit spontaneous desynchrony between circadian and sleep:wake cycles occurs when they are allowed to self-select their wake:sleep and light:dark schedules.[37] Under these conditions, the observed cycle length usually is longer than the endogenous circadian pacemaker's period of approximately 24.2 hours,[38] and there is no longer the opportunity to study all possible timing combinations of circadian and homeostatic factors. The observed circadian period also is approximately 25 hours instead of approximately 24.2 hours; this apparent discrepancy can be explained by the nonuniform (across the day) light exposure,[39] such that there is more light exposure during the circadian phases that cause phase delays. Nevertheless, spontaneous desynchrony protocols have also yielded much useful information on the effects of circadian rhythmicity and sleep homeostasis on sleep.[40]

EFFECTS OF SELF-SELECTED BEHAVIORS ON CIRCADIAN RHYTHMS AND SLEEP

There also are direct and indirect effects of behaviors that may affect both circadian rhythmicity and sleep homeostasis (**Fig. 3**). Light during the normal dark times can

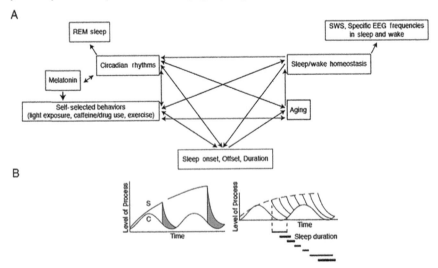

Fig. 3. The regulation of sleep and wake. (A) Inter-relationships of factors affecting multiple aspects of sleep and wake. (B). Diagrams of changes in time of (left) two-process model of sleep regulation. S, process S, the sleep homeostatic factor; C, process C, the circadian rhythm process; gray areas, time of sleep. When an individual self-selects sleep onset (1 of the 2 vertical lines), the level of homeostatic drive is at the process S level (upper line); homeostatic drive then declines in an exponential manner until it reaches the process C level. Then the person awakens and the level of homeostatic drive begins to rise again (not shown). (Right) Sleep durations associated with different self-selected sleep onsets.

induce sleep in rodents, and dark during the normal light times can induce wake. In addition, as described previously, self-selected light:dark timing may affect alertness and circadian rhythms, which then affect timing of sleep (which occurs in the dark). Self-selected light:dark timing differentially affects early lark versus late owl chronotypes and their circadian phase. When larks and owls can choose their own lighting schedules, circadian phase is later in owls than larks; but when all are exposed to the same light:dark schedule, circadian phase is approximately the same in all.[41] Caffeine can directly affect the circadian system[42] as well as increase alertness, which then includes increased light that can directly affect the circadian clock.

Self-selected light:dark schedules may be involved in some circadian rhythm sleep disorders. For example, individuals who do not choose regular light:dark schedules or live mostly under indoor dim light conditions, blind people, or individuals with relatively long endogenous periods who stay up late at night or for long durations (possibly because of endogenous induced or pharmaceutically induced low sleep homeostatic pressure buildup rate) and have light exposure that promotes circadian delays may develop non–24-hour sleep:wake disorder (see Abbott, this issue). Or, individuals with reduced light sensitivity or preferential late-night light exposure may develop delayed sleep phase syndrome (see Wyatt and Culnan, this issue). A reduced rate of rise of sleep homeostatic pressure (as postulated to occur with aging) would affect the relative amplitudes of circadian and homeostatic influences on sleep timing, and, together with a relative circadian phase advance, may be a reason for early morning awakening complaints of many older people.

MARKERS OF CIRCADIAN RHYTHMS IN HUMANS

Circadian rhythms generated by the SCN heavily influence the timing of sleep onset and offset and of the timing of REM sleep within a sleep episode. The SCN's tight regulation of melatonin rhythmicity (discussed previously) makes melatonin a valuable marker of circadian timing if melatonin is collected under dim light conditions, because ocular light exposure suppresses melatonin. Another marker of circadian timing and amplitude is CBT; however, given the circadian phase–dependent masking effects of sleep:wake and activity on CBT, it cannot be used as a marker of circadian phase and amplitude except under highly controlled inpatient conditions. Melatonin (usually dim light melatonin onset [DLMO]) and CBT (usually minimum of fit sinusoidal curve [CBT_{min}]) markers are tightly linked in both phase (ie, DLMO occurring approximately 6 hours before CBT_{min}[43]) and amplitude.[38,44,45] Unexpectedly, even though melatonin levels are high when individuals are usually tired, it is not effective as a hypnotic[46] when taken for insomnia and/or at an individual's habitual sleep time. On the other hand, melatonin or its agonists can phase shift the circadian pacemaker of sighted and blind people[47,48] and through that mechanism affect sleep. That sleep itself can modulate pacemaker function already has been noted earlier in this review[16]; sleep restriction also can decrease the effectiveness of phase-shifting light stimuli,[49] an interaction that may be important for some circadian rhythm sleep disorders.

CIRCADIAN AND HOMEOSTATIC EFFECTS ON SLEEP

Paradoxically, in humans, the circadian drive for sleep is strongest near the end of the habitual sleep episode, perhaps to consolidate sleep as the homeostatic drive decreases during the sleep episode, whereas the circadian drive for wake is strongest a few hours before habitual sleep during the wake maintenance zone, perhaps to consolidate wake as sleep homeostatic drive builds up over an approximately 16-hour wake episode.[50] REM sleep is most likely to occur during the end of the habitual sleep episode, both because that is the time the circadian drive promotes REM sleep and because the NREM-REM sleep competition across the night has decreased NREM sleep pressure as sleep homeostasis declines.

The timing and content of sleep, including sleep latency and wake within a sleep episode, are regulated by a nonlinear interaction between these circadian and sleep homeostatic processes: the magnitude of the circadian influence depends on how long an individual has been awake or asleep. When a person has just awoken, there is little circadian variation in sleep latency; similarly, when a person has just fallen asleep, there is little circadian variation in wake within a sleep episode. If the person has been awake for a long time, however, then sleep latency depends on circadian phase (large-amplitude circadian influence); and if the person has been asleep for a long time, then the amount of wake within the sleep episode depends on circadian phase. Therefore, when sleep homeostasis and circadian phase are aligned, there is relatively short sleep latency and consolidated sleep without significant wake within the sleep episodes.[50] The two, however, are misaligned in jet lag and shift work; during these conditions, the circadian system is promoting sleep when the individual desires to be awake and promoting wake when the individual desires to be asleep. The nonlinear combination of sleep homeostasis and circadian phase also affects some EEG frequencies[51] and cortical and subcortical activity in the brain as measured by functional MRI.[52]

CODA

Circadian neurobiology and sleep:wake regulation affect virtually all physiologic systems, including each other. Self-selected behaviors also may affect these processes, leading to cycles that may cause diseases or disorders (eg, jet lag, shift work, and/or other circadian rhythm sleep disorders) and influence multiple physiologic, metabolic, immunologic, and mental functions. Understanding the underlying physiology is crucial for developing and testing appropriate educational, behavioral, pharmaceutical, and other interventions to lessen these adverse consequences.

REFERENCES

1. Dunlap JC, Loros JJ, DeCoursey PJ, editors. Chronobiology: biological time-keeping. Sunderland (MA): Sinauer Associates; 2009. p. 382.
2. Roenneberg T, Merrow M. The circadian clock and human health. Curr Biol 2016; 26:R432-43.
3. Paul MJ, Zucker I, Schwartz WJ. Tracking the seasons: the internal calendars of animals. Philos Trans R Soc Lond B Biol Sci 2008;363:341-61.
4. Wood S, Loudon A. Clocks for all seasons: unwinding the roles and mechanisms of circadian and interval timers in the hypothalamus and pituitary. J Endocrinol 2014;222:R39-59.
5. Wever RA. Internal interactions within the human circadian system: the masking effect. Experientia 1985;41:332-42.
6. Helm B, Visser ME, Schwartz WJ, et al. Two sides of a coin: ecological and chronobiological perspectives of timing in the wild. Philos Trans R Soc Lond B Biol Sci 2017;372:20160246.
7. Roenneberg T, Wirz-Justice A, Merrow M. Life between clocks: daily temporal patterns of human chronotypes. J Biol Rhythms 2003;18:80-90.
8. Takahashi JS. Transcriptional architecture of the mammalian circadian clock. Nat Rev Genet 2017;18:164-79.

9. Mohawk JA, Green CB, Takahashi JS. Central and peripheral circadian clocks in mammals. Annu Rev Neurosci 2012;35:445–62.
10. Schibler U, Gotic I, Saini C, et al. Clock-talk: interactions between central and peripheral circadian oscillators in mammals. Cold Spring Harb Symp Quant Biol 2015;80:223–32.
11. Lamia KA, Storch K-F, Weitz CJ. Physiological significance of a peripheral tissue circadian clock. Proc Natl Acad Sci U S A 2008;105:15172–7.
12. Qian J, Scheer FAJL. Circadian system and glucose metabolism: implications for physiology and disease. Trends Endocrinol Metab 2016;27:282–93.
13. Yamazaki S, Yoshikawa T, Biscoe EW, et al. Ontogeny of circadian organization in the rat. J Biol Rhythms 2009;24:55–63.
14. Weaver DR. The suprachiasmatic nucleus: a 25-year retrospective. J Biol Rhythms 1998;13:100–12.
15. Houben T, Coomans CP, Meijer JH. Regulation of circadian and acute activity levels by the murine suprachiasmatic nuclei. PLoS One 2014;9:e110172.
16. Deboer T, Vansteensel MJ, Détári L, et al. Sleep states alter activity of suprachiasmatic nucleus neurons. Nat Neurosci 2003;6:1086–90.
17. Ralph MR, Foster RG, Davis FC, et al. Transplanted suprachiasmatic nucleus determines circadian period. Science 1990;247:975–8.
18. LeGates TA, Fernandez DC, Hattar S. Light as a central modulator of circadian rhythms, sleep and affect. Nat Rev Neurosci 2014;15:443–54.
19. Mistlberger RE. Circadian regulation of sleep in mammals: role of the suprachiasmatic nucleus. Brain Res Rev 2005;49:429–54.
20. Saper CB, Scammell TE, Lu J. Hypothalamic regulation of sleep and circadian rhythms. Nature 2005;437:1257–63.
21. Smale L, Lee T, Nunez AA. Mammalian diurnality: some facts and gaps. J Biol Rhythms 2003;18:356–66.
22. Kramer A, Yang FC, Snodgrass P, et al. Regulation of daily locomotor activity and sleep by hypothalamic EGF receptor signaling. Science 2001;294:2511–5.
23. Zhou QY, Cheng MY. Prokineticin 2 and circadian clock output. FEBS J 2005;272:5703–9.
24. Welsh DK, Takahashi JS, Kay SA. Suprachiasmatic nucleus: cell autonomy and network properties. Annu Rev Physiol 2010;72:551–77.
25. Hastings MH, Maywood ES, Brancaccio M. Generation of circadian rhythms in the suprachiasmatic nucleus. Nat Rev Neurosci 2018;19:453–69.
26. Brown EN, Lydic R, Schiff ND. General anesthesia, sleep, and coma. N Engl J Med 2010;363:2638–50.
27. Saper CB, Fuller PM. Wake-sleep circuitry: an overview. Curr Opin Neurobiol 2017;44:186–92.
28. Scammell TE, Arrigoni, Lipton JO. Neural circuitry of wakefulness and sleep. Neuron 2017;93:747–65.
29. Everson CA. Functional consequences of sustained sleep deprivation in the rat. Behav Brain Res 1995;69:43–54.
30. Available at: https://www.nytimes.com/2007/10/23/science/23quot.html. Accessed April 8, 2019.
31. Borbély AA. A two process model of sleep regulation. Hum Neurobiol 1982;1:195–204.
32. Aeschbach D, Matthews JR, Postolache TT, et al. Dynamics of the human EEG during prolonged wakefulness: evidence for frequency-specific circadian and homeostatic influences. Neurosci Lett 1997;239:121–4.

33. Cohen DA, Wang W, Wyatt JK, et al. Uncovering residual effects of chronic sleep loss on human performance. Sci Transl Med 2010;2:14ra13.
34. Phillips AJK, Klerman EB, Butler JP. Modeling the adenosine system as a modulator of cognitive performance and sleep patterns during sleep restriction and recovery. PLoS Comput Biol 2017;12:e1005759.
35. Carskadon MA, Dement WC. Sleep studies on a 90-minute day. Electroencephalogr Clin Neurophysiol 1975;39:145–55.
36. McHill AW, Hull JT, Wang W, et al. Chronic sleep curtailment, even without extended (>16 h) wakefulness, degrades human vigilance performance. Proc Natl Acad Sci U S A 2018;115:6070–5.
37. Wever RA. The circadian system of man: results of experiments under temporal isolation. New York: Springer-Verlag; 1979. p. 276.
38. Duffy JF, Cain SW, Chang AM, et al. Sex difference in the near-24-hour intrinsic period of the human circadian timing system. Proc Natl Acad Sci U S A 2011; 108:15602–8.
39. Klerman EB, Dijk DJ, Kronauer RE, et al. Simulations of light effects on the human circadian pacemaker: implications for assessment of intrinsic period. Am J Physiol 1996;270:R271–82.
40. Strogatz SH, Kronauer RE, Czeisler CA. Circadian regulation dominates homeostatic control of sleep length and prior wake length in humans. Sleep 1986;9:353–64.
41. Wright KP Jr, McHill AW, Birks BR, et al. Entrainment of the human circadian clock to the natural light-dark cycle. Curr Biol 2013;23:1554–8.
42. Burke TM, Markwald RR, McHill AW, et al. Effects of caffeine on the human circadian clock in vivo and in vitro. Sci Transl Med 2015;7:305ra146.
43. Dahl K, Avery DH, Lewy AJ, et al. Dim light melatonin onset and circadian temperature during a constant routine in hypersomnia winter depression. Acta Psychiatr Scand 1993;88:60–6.
44. Shanahan TL, Czeisler CA. Light exposure induces equivalent phase shifts of the endogenous circadian rhythms of circulating plasma melatonin and core body temperature in men. J Clin Endocrinol Metab 1991;73:227–35.
45. Shanahan TL, Kronauer RE, Duffy JF, et al. Melatonin rhythms observed throughout a three-cycle bright-light stimulus designed to reset the human circadian pacemaker. J Biol Rhythms 1999;14:237–53.
46. Sateia MJ, Buysse DJ, Krystal AD, et al. Clinical practice guideline for the pharmacologic treatment of chronic insomnia in adults: an American Academy of Sleep Medicine clinical practice guideline. J Clin Sleep Med 2017;13:307–49.
47. Rajaratnam SM, Polymeropoulos MH, Fisher DM, et al. Melatonin agonist tasimelteon (VEC162) for transient insomnia after sleep-time shift: two randomised controlled multicenter trials. Lancet 2008;373:482–91.
48. Lockley SW, Skene DJ, James K, et al. Melatonin administration can entrain the free running circadian system of blind subjects. J Endocrinol 2000;164:R1–6.
49. Burgess HJ. Partial sleep deprivation reduces phase advances to light in humans. J Biol Rhythms 2010;25:460–8.
50. Dijk DJ, Czeisler CA. Paradoxical timing of the circadian rhythm of sleep propensity serves to consolidate sleep and wakefulness in humans. Neurosci Lett 1994; 166:63–8.
51. Dijk DJ, Czeisler CA. Contribution of the circadian pacemaker and the sleep homeostat to sleep propensity, sleep structure, electroencephalographic slow waves, and sleep spindle activity in humans. J Neurosci 1995;15:3526–38.
52. Muto V, Jaspar M, Meyer C, et al. Local modulation of human brain responses by circadian rhythmicity and sleep debt. Science 2016;353:687–90.

Genetics of Circadian Rhythms

Martha Hotz Vitaterna, PhD[a,b],*, Kazuhiro Shimomura, DVM, PhD[a,c],
Peng Jiang, PhD[a,b]

KEYWORDS

- Circadian rhythms • Polymorphisms • Patterns of gene activity • Clock genes

KEY POINTS

- Circadian rhythms are generated by a genetic mechanism: a feedback loop of gene transcription and translation of core "clock genes." This genetic clock mechanism functions in diverse cell and tissue types throughout the body.
- Genetic polymorphisms in both core clock genes and interacting genes contribute to individual differences in the expression and properties of circadian rhythms.
- The circadian clock profoundly influences the patterns of gene activity in diverse tissues, indicating a mechanism by which it that can influence the expression and development of disease.

INTRODUCTION: THE MANY LEVELS OF CIRCADIAN GENETICS

The topic, "Genetics of Circadian Rhythms," could be a consideration of several questions. Are differences between individuals in their circadian rhythmicity a result of differences in their genes? If so, what genes? What genes encode the "clock" mechanism? How can genes form a clock? Does the circadian clock mechanism affect gene activity? If so, how?

Here, the authors describe the developing appreciation of the multiple interconnections of circadian rhythmicity with genetics in mammals. As illustrated in **Fig. 1**, a core set of genes functions as a clock in every cell as a feedback loop of gene transcription and translation: providing a means for circadian rhythms to persist independently in each cell. However, the clocks within the cell can be influenced by a variety of interacting pathways and influences ranging from the intracellular (eg, redox state) to nutritional, endocrine, and behavioral. Similarly, a variety of genetic polymorphisms in other genes appear to influence the expression of circadian rhythms in individuals. The genetic

 a Center for Sleep and Circadian Biology; b Department of Neurobiology, Weinberg College of Arts and Sciences, Northwestern University, 2205 Tech Drive, Evanston, IL 60208, USA; c Davee Department of Neurology, Feinberg School of Medicine, Northwestern University, 420 East Superior Street, Chicago, IL 60611, USA
* Corresponding author. Northwestern University, Center for Sleep and Circadian Biology, 2205 Tech Drive, Evanston, IL 60208.
E-mail address: m-vitaterna@northwestern.edu

Neurol Clin 37 (2019) 487–504
https://doi.org/10.1016/j.ncl.2019.05.002
0733-8619/19/© 2019 Elsevier Inc. All rights reserved.

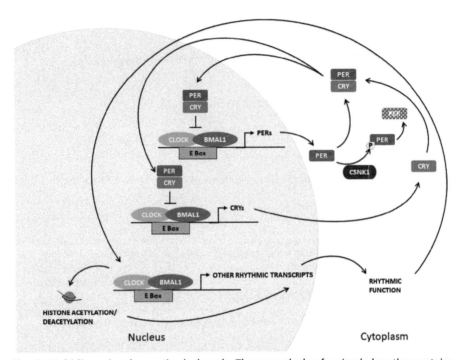

Fig. 1. Multidimensional genetic clockwork. The core clock of animals has the proteins CLOCK and BMAL1 functioning as positive regulators, binding to E-box regulatory elements and transactivating the transcription of the *per* and *Cry* genes as well as multiple other rhythmically expressed genes. Phosphorylation of PER by CSNK1 can lead to its degradation. PER and CRY proteins form dimers and enter the nucleus to repress the CLOCK:BMAL1 complex. Rhythmic transcription leads to rhythms in key regulator genes and cellular functions that can feedback to alter core clock function. In addition, CLOCK affects histone acetylation, another mechanism by which gene activity can be modulated.

circadian clock regulates rhythms of gene expression via direct transcriptional regulation, and histone acetylation/deacetylation. Despite the many genes and mechanisms, such results point to a very central role of circadian clock genes in regulating biochemical, metabolic, and physiologic processes at many different levels of organization.

CIRCADIAN RHYTHMS ARE HERITABLE

One of the first questions to consider is one of "Nature or Nurture." To what extent are attributes of circadian rhythms determined by one's genes (Nature) as opposed to one's environment (Nurture)? A variety of experimental approaches to this question have been used over the years, all supporting the role of genetics. For example, attempts to alter the endogenous period of mice by gestation and rearing under non-24-hour days (either 20-hour or 28-hour light-dark cycles) failed to have lasting effects on the free-running period in the mice as adults.[1] Mice of an inbred strain, which are effectively genetically identical to one another, but genetically distinct from mice of another strain, can be compared. Significant differences between strains in circadian rhythm properties have been noted,[2–6] that are above and beyond the differences between individuals of the same strain.

Similarly, studies of human twins have provided a means to estimate the "heritability" (proportion of phenotypic variance attributable to genetic variance) of circadian rhythms. The extent to which monozygotic (identical) twins are more similar than dizygotic twins can be used to estimate heritability. Hence, significant heritability has been described for the timing and pattern of serum cortisol rhythms[7,8] and of chronotype (morningness vs eveningness)[9,10] by twin comparisons.

Evidence of heritability does not provide an indication of the number or identity of the genes at play, however. Genes contributing to 1 aspect of circadian rhythmicity (the endogenous or "free-running" periodicity, for example) may be different from those involved in another (such as morning vs evening preference). Furthermore, variants in genes involved in critical functions may be deleterious and thus eliminated by natural selection, meaning that the allelic polymorphisms naturally present in populations (and represented in strain or twin comparisons) may be in different genes from those essential for generation of circadian timing. Hence, there are many reasons to expect the existence of multiple types of circadian rhythm genes.

THE CORE CIRCADIAN CLOCK

Early evidence suggested a genetic mechanism lay at the core generator of self-sustained circadian rhythms. In 1961, Colin Pittendrigh[11] noted that the clock mechanism could be contained in single cells and was considered unlikely to be simply a chemical reaction because it was relatively insensitive to being sped up or slowed down by changes in temperature. Further evidence that gene transcription and translation were involved included demonstration that inhibition of protein synthesis could reset, or temporarily stop, the circadian clock.[12-14] To identify what the genes and proteins comprising the circadian clock were, induction of mutations and screening for abnormal circadian rhythms proved the most effective approach, in both *Drosophila melanogaster*[15] and in mice.[16] Mutagenesis and phenotypic screening has also been successful in identifying circadian clock genes in other organisms, such as the fungus *Neurospora crassa*,[17] plants,[18] and cyanobacteria.[19]

The identification of the transcription-translation feedback genes now known to form the core circadian clock are described here. The "positive" elements CLOCK and BMAL1 drive the transcription of the "negative" elements PER and CRY, that in turn feedback to inhibit CLOCK:BMAL1.

Period

The first identified clock component gene, *period* (denoted *per*), was discovered in 1971 in *Drosophila* by a "forward genetic" approach consisting of chemically inducing random mutations in the genome, and detecting those mutations that affect circadian rhythms by screening the progeny of the mutagenized individuals for altered rhythmicity.[15] This approach has the advantage that no assumptions are made about the nature of the genes or gene products involved, but is based on the presumption that there exist single genes that, when mutated, will alter rhythms in a detectable manner. At the time, this presumption of the existence of single genes that could regulate a complex behavior was considered radical or absurd, but now appears to have been foresight.

Initially, 3 alleles of the *per* gene were identified by the process of mutagenesis and screening. Flies carrying these alleles had either no apparent rhythm in eclosion (emergence from the pupal case) or locomotion, or had either long (approximately 29 hours) or short periods (approximately 19 hours) for the rhythms of eclosion and locomotor activity.[15]

Confirmation of the importance of the *per* gene as a central circadian clock component was possible upon its molecular identification, for which the 2017 Nobel Prize was awarded to Hall, Rosbash, and Young. The gene's function was demonstrated by rescue of the arrhythmic mutant phenotype after introduction of the wild-type allele of the *per* gene into mutant flies.[20–22] The level of the messenger RNA (mRNA) transcript encoded by the *per* gene was shown to oscillate in a circadian fashion [40] as a result of transcriptional regulation,[23] and the levels of the PER protein were shown to lag the *per* mRNA levels.[24] In fact, shifts in the circadian phase can be evoked by the induction of PER protein under the control of a noncircadian promoter.[25] Thus, many lines of evidence indicate that the *per* gene encodes a protein that is a clock component. Three orthologs of the *per* gene, *Per1*, *Per2*, and *Per3*, have now been identified in mammals, and the levels of their mRNA have also been shown to oscillate with a circadian period.[26–30]

Clock

In the early 1990s, no genes in mammals had been identified as even possible candidate circadian clock genes, leading to an effort to again apply chemical mutagenesis and phenotypic screening, this time in mice. In a screen of more than 300 first-generation progeny of mutagen-treated mice (potential heterozygous mutants), Vitaterna and colleagues[16] found 1 animal that had a free-running period of about 24.8 hours, more than 6 standard deviations longer than the mean of about 24.7 hours. In homozygotes, this mutation results in a dramatic lengthening of the period to about 28 hours, which is usually followed by the eventual loss of circadian rhythmicity (ie, arrhythmicity) after about 1 to 3 weeks in constant darkness. The affected gene was named *Clock* (an acronym for *Circadian locomotor output cycles kaput*[16]) and mapped to mouse chromosome 5.[16,31] The *Clock* gene was cloned by a combination of genetic rescue and positional cloning. *Clock/Clock* mutant mice were phenotypically rescued by a bacterial artificial chromosome transgene that contained the *Clock* gene, allowing for functional identification of the gene.[32] The *Clock* gene encodes a transcriptional regulatory protein having a basic helix-loop-helix DNA-binding domain, a PAS dimerization domain, and a Q-rich transactivation domain. The mutant form of the CLOCK protein (CLOCK-Δ19) lacks a portion of the activation domain found in wild-type protein, and thus, although it is capable of protein dimerization, transcriptional activation is diminished or lost. The protein dimerization domain is named PAS because the genes originally identified with it were, *per*, *ARNT*, and *sim*. *Clock* mRNA is expressed in the suprachiasmatic nuclei (SCN) as well as other tissues, but it does not oscillate in a circadian manner in all tissues.[33]

Bmal1

The presence of the PAS dimerization domain in CLOCK protein led to a screen for potential partners for the CLOCK protein. A protein of unknown function, BMAL1 (Brain and Muscle ARNT-Like 1, now denoted ARNT-Like or *Arntl*), was able to dimerize with the CLOCK protein.[34] Creation of mice with a null allele of *Bmal1* demonstrated the critical role of this gene in circadian rhythm generation. These mutant mice, although displaying light-dark responsive differences in activity level, become arrhythmic immediately upon release in constant darkness.

Additional actions of the CLOCK:BMAL1 heterodimer have become clear. Although *Clock* mRNA does not oscillate, its protein's nuclear versus cytoplasmic localization does.[35] By studying the intracellular localization of CLOCK and BMAL1 in fibroblasts of mouse embryos with mutations in different clock genes, and ectopically expressing the proteins, it was found that nuclear accumulation of CLOCK was dependent on formation of the CLOCK:BMAL1 dimer, as was phosphorylation of the complex and its degradation.[35] Other PAS domain-containing proteins failed to affect the localization of CLOCK, indicating that these posttranslational events are specific to the CLOCK:-BMAL1 dimer.

Following the identification of CLOCK:BMAL1 dimerization, the ability of this heterodimer to regulate transcription was tested using a reporter construct based on the upstream regulatory elements of the *per* gene. The *per* gene of *Drosophila* contains an upstream regulatory element, the "clock control region," within which is contained a sequence needed for positive regulation of transcription, the E-box element (CACGTG).[36] CLOCK-BMAL1 heterodimers were found to activate transcription of *Per* genes in a process that requires binding to the E-box element.[34] However, CLOCK-Δ19 mutant protein was not able to activate transcription, consistent with the finding that exon 19, which is skipped in *Clock* mutants,[33] is necessary for transactivation. Thus, CLOCK protein interacts with the regulatory regions of the *per* gene to allow transcription of the *per* mRNA and eventual translation of PER protein. However, this positive regulation alone will not produce an oscillation in *per* mRNA levels, which is known to be responsible for the oscillation in PER protein levels.[23] Findings that the *Clock* mutation dramatically decreases *per* genes' expression also confirms the positive regulation of CLOCK:BMAL1 on *per* transcription in situ.[37,38] Mice with null mutations of *Per1*, *Per2*, or *Per3* alone display altered circadian periods,[39,40] whereas mice with both *Per1* and *Per2* null mutations lose rhythmicity. *Per3* null mutant mice exhibit only a subtle alteration in rhythmicity and *Per1/Per3* or *Per2/Per3* double mutants are not substantially distinct from the *Per1* or *Per2* single mutants. These findings suggest there may be some functional redundancy among the different mammalian *per* genes, but raise the question of the role of *Per3* in mammalian circadian rhythms.

Cryptochromes

Cryptochromes are blue light–responsive flavoprotein photopigments related to photolyases, so named because their function was cryptic when first identified. In mammals, 2 cryptochrome genes, *Cry1* and *Cry2*, have been identified and were found to be highly expressed in the ganglion cells and inner nuclear layer of the retina as well as the SCN,[41] and their mRNA expression levels oscillate in these tissues. Targeted mutant mice lacking *Cry2* exhibit a lengthened circadian period, whereas mice lacking *Cry1* have a shortened circadian period; mice with both mutations have immediate loss of rhythmicity upon transfer to constant darkness.[42–45] Thus, like the mammalian *period* genes, the *cryptochrome* genes appear to have both distinct (given their opposite effects on circadian period) and compensatory (given that either gene can sustain rhythmicity in the absence of the other) functions.

Further evidence for a central clock function is the finding that the *cryptochromes* appear to share several regulatory features with the *period* genes. In *Clock* mutant mice, the mRNA levels of *Cry1* and *Cry2* are reduced in the SCN and in skeletal muscle,[46] suggesting that the *cryptochromes* also are induced by CLOCK:BMAL1 transactivation. Using mammalian cell lines, CRY1 and CRY2 were found by coimmunoprecipitation to interact with PER1, PER2, and PER3, leading to nuclear localization of the CRY:PER dimer as indicated by cotransfection assays with epitope-tagged proteins.[46] Either CRY:CRY or CRY:PER complexes were capable of inhibiting CLOCK:BMAL1 transactivation of *Per1* or vasopressin transcription.[46] Thus, the CRYs as well as the PERs are capable of a negative feedback function, inhibiting CLOCK:BMAL1-induced transcription.

Casein Kinase 1

The *tau* mutation of the hamster arose spontaneously in a laboratory stock.[47] The mutation is semidominant and shortens the period from 24 to 22 hours in heterozygotes, and 20 hours in homozygotes. The mutation predated the *Clock* mutation and demonstrated that single-gene mutations could profoundly alter[48] the circadian clock in mammals, just as in flies and *Neurospora*. Unfortunately, the genetic tools needed for cloning this important and interesting gene were not available for the hamster, and thus, its molecular identity could not be determined by conventional genetic mapping/positional cloning approaches.

Lowrey and colleagues[49] were able to identify a genomic region of conserved synteny (a grouping of genes together on a chromosome) in hamsters, mice, and humans that encompassed the *tau* mutation. *Tau* was thus identified as being a mutation in the *Casein Kinase 1 epsilon* (*CK1e*) gene, the mammalian ortholog of the *Drosophila doubletime* gene. Sequencing of the gene identified a point mutation, which leads to altered enzyme dynamics and autophosphorylation state. CK1e can phosphorylate PER proteins, and the *tau* mutant enzyme is deficient in this ability. Thus, CK1e may lead to degradation of PERs, slowing the accumulation of PER in the nucleus and thus repression of CLOCK:BMAL1. *Casein Kinase 1 delta* (*CK1d*) has also been implicated in mammalian circadian rhythmicity.[50–53]

INTERACTING CLOCK PATHWAYS

Although not depicted in **Fig. 1**, several genes have been identified as key regulators of the core circadian clock genes. These genes form additional feedback loops to the genetic clock and are described here.

Rev-Erb Alpha and ROR

Although the negative feedback of PER and CRY proteins on their own CLOCK:BMAL1-induced transcription constitutes a form of negative feedback and may be sufficient to explain the oscillations in expression of *Per* and *Cry* genes, the rhythmic expression of *Bmal1* with an opposite phase was not explained by this feedback. *Rev-erbα*, an orphan nuclear receptor (now denoted *Nr1d1*), was the missing link. Its promoter region contains 3 E-boxes, and transcription is thus positively regulated by CLOCK and BMAL1.[54] Its transcription is negatively regulated by PER and CRYs and is at a minimum when mPER2 is at a maximum, and it is constitutively expressed at intermediate levels in *Cry1/Cry2* or *Per1/Per2* double knockouts. REV-ERBα protein appears to drive the circadian oscillation in *Bmal1* transcription: the *Bmal1* promoter includes 2 RORE sequences (enhancer sequences that recognize members of the REV-ERB and ROR orphan nuclear receptor families), and *Bmal1* expression is drastically reduced in *Rev-erba* null mutants.[54] Thus *Rev-erbα* may act to link the positive and negative regulatory signals of other clock genes to the transcription of *Bmal1* and to cellular metabolism. CLOCK:BMAL1 activity is suppressed by an NAD^+-dependent deacetylase SIRT1, which is in turn regulated by the circadian control of NAD^+ biosynthesis.[55–58]

Rev-erba also contributes to the differences between the phase of *Cry1* mRNA rhythms relative to other clock genes, whose transcription is enhanced by CLOCK:BMAL binding to E-boxes. The *Cry1* gene has 3 candidate REV-ERB/ROR binding sites[59]; in vitro assays indicate that REV-ERBα binds to 2 of these sites. Luciferase reporter assays indicate that REV-ERBα protein can inhibit transcription of *Cry1* through binding at these 2 sites. REV-ERBβ also appears to share some functional redundancy with REV-ERBα.[60]

Fbxl3 and Fbxl21

In addition to *Rev-erb*, other genes modulate the *Cryptochromes*. The *Overtime* mutation in mice was identified in a mutagenesis screen based on a lengthened free-running circadian period.[61] The responsible mutation was ultimately identified as being in a known gene encoding the F-box protein *Fbxl3*, but a gene previously unknown to be involved in circadian rhythmicity. *Fbxl3^{OVTM}* mutant appears to be functionally comparable to null mutants. FBXL3 protein leads to degradation of CRY1, whereas the FBXL3-OVTM mutant protein is less effective in this capacity. Thus, the period lengthening may be a direct result of a delay in degradation of CRY, effectively preventing the core cycle from restarting. The closely related protein FBXL21[62] has been found to function in a similar manner.[63,64]

NPAS2

NPAS2 (neuronal PAS family member 2) shares the closest homology with CLOCK of all identified bHLH-PAS family members. Null mutants of this gene have altered circadian activity patterns, notably the absence of a "siesta" in later subjective night, but no dramatic alterations in circadian free-running period or persistence.[65] However, when null mutants of the *Clock* had less dramatic phenotypes than the dominant-negative Δ19 mutant,[31,66] the role of NPAS2 was reexamined. In the absence of functioning CLOCK, NPAS2 appears to be able to partially compensate.[67]

Dec1 and Dec2

Like other clock genes, *Dec1* and *Dec2* are basic helix-loop-helix transcription factors that bind to E-boxes. DEC1 and DEC2 have been found to inhibit transactivation of *Per* by CLOCK and BMAL1.[68] DEC1 and DEC2 form dimers.[69] The inhibition of CLOCK and BMAL1 transactivation may be related to interactions with BMAL1, but can also be attributed to binding to (and thus possibly competition for) E-boxes.[70] A human allelic variant in *Dec2* has been linked with total sleep time.[71] This functional relationship has been confirmed in transgenic mice expressing the human *Dec2* allele.

POLYGENIC CIRCADIAN TRAITS

A few spontaneous allelic variants in core clock genes have been identified from a familial pattern that suggests a single gene pattern of inheritance. For example, a familial form of Delayed Sleep Wake Phase Disorder (the most common circadian sleepwake disorder) has been identified, associated with a mutation in the *CRY1* gene.[72] There is a strong familial component to Advanced Sleep Wake Phase Disorder (ASWPD)[73], with mutations demonstrated in *casein kinase Id*,[51] and the *casein kinase Ie* binding region of *PER2*[74] and of *CRY2*.[75] These mutations result in a more rapid progression through the transcription/translation feedback loop, leading to an overall shorter intrinsic circadian period.[76] However, in most cases, traits such as intrinsic circadian period are continuous or quantitative (rather than discrete or qualitative), indicative of multiple genetic loci influencing the trait.

Two general approaches to the identification of genes underlying heritability of circadian rhythms in mammals have been taken. In mice, the approach of identification of quantitative trait loci (QTLs) uses linkage mapping to find genes or genomic regions that contribute to quantitative differences in circadian traits. In humans, the approach of Genome-Wide Association Studies (GWAS) uses statistical association of circadian phenotypic traits to genetic polymorphisms in populations.

Quantitative Trait Loci

Genetic heterogeneity underlies many phenotypic variations observed in circadian rhythmicity. The complex nature of circadian behavior is reflected in the phenotypic variability observed in mammalian species; this has been described particularly well in mice. Significant differences in circadian behavior have been demonstrated when comparing multiple inbred strains of mice.[2–5] In particular, when the endogenous period has been measured, differences of nearly a full hour have been observed among the most divergent strains. Strain differences are also present in other aspects of circadian behavior, including entrainment to light-dark cycles and the robustness of the rhythm. Crosses among such inbred strains have indicated a polygenic basis for these differences in circadian behavior.

The first comprehensive QTL analysis of circadian behavior in mammals (mouse) and the first to use genetic interaction analysis to identify QTLs was conducted in 2001.[77] In this work, 14 QTLs in the mouse genome associated with 5 different phenotypic traits underlying circadian behavior. Importantly, all but one of these QTLs did *not* overlap with known circadian clock genes, demonstrating that many allelic variants in genes beyond the canonical circadian clock mechanism must exist. Although severe disruption of circadian rhythms may be caused by mutations in core clock genes, it is possible that the broad variety of circadian behavior observed in mammalian species, including humans, are the result of polymorphisms in multiple, interacting loci.

Molecular identification of interacting quantitative trait loci

Quantitative genetic approaches were used to identify modifiers of the original *Clock* mutation, *Clock^{Δ19}*, in the genetic backgrounds of C3H/HeJ and BALB/cJ inbred mouse strains. In C3H/HeJ, genetic suppression of circadian phenotype in *Clock^{Δ19}* mutant mice is mediated via the melatonin biosynthetic pathway.[78] Two major QTLs were mapped on chromosomes 11 and X in which genes encoding melatonin biosynthetic enzymes, *Aanat* (arylakylamine N-acetyltransferase) and *Asmt* (acetylserotonin O-methyltransferase), are mapped, respectively. It has been known that most laboratory mouse strains, except C3H/HeJ and CBA/J, do not make a detectable level of melatonin due to the mutations on *Aanat* and *Asmt*.[79,80] Melatonin and the selective melatonin agonist, ramelteon, indeed can phenocopy the genetic suppression of the *Clock^{Δ19}* mutation in the SCN. The *Clock^{Δ19}* mutation has also been shown to be associated with metabolic syndrome in mice.[81] It is therefore interesting that the melatonin receptor 1B (*MTNR1B*) gene has been strongly associated with fasting serum glucose levels in humans.[82–84] Perhaps the suppressive effects of melatonin on circadian rhythm may also have relevance to other phenotypes, such as metabolism.

On the other hand, the gene responsible for suppression of the *Clock^{Δ19}* mutant phenotypic in the BALB/cJ strain background is a transcription factor, *Usf1*. Phenotypic suppression occurs as a consequence of a single-nucleotide change in the promoter region that increases mRNA and protein expression in BALB/cJ mice.[85] USF1 and CLOCK:BMAL1 compete for the same E-box regulatory sites in circadian genes, such as *Per1*, *Per2*, or *Dbp*. The *Clock^{Δ19}* mutation significantly reduces the affinity of CLOCK:-BMAL1 binding to E-box sites. The reduced affinity of the mutant CLOCK:BMAL1 complex permits USF1 to compete more effectively for the same E-box sites, and the transcriptional activation potential of USF1 can then rescue the reduced transcriptional activation of the CLOCKΔ19 mutant protein. USF1 and CLOCK:BMAL1 DNA binding were examined on a genome-wide basis using ChIP-Seq technology. The *Clock^{Δ19}* mutant causes dramatic increases in USF1 binding genome-wide and also reveals that the USF1 and CLOCK:BMAL1 transcriptional networks interact extensively. The interactions have ramifications for understanding the shared role of USF1 and CLOCK:BMAL1 in the regulation of metabolism and lipid biosynthetic pathways.

Genome-Wide Association Studies

GWAS are used to identify associations between chromosomal regions (loci) and trait of interest in human. Because genomic regions of linkage disequilibrium are much smaller in human populations (<100 kb) than in experimental mouse cross (40–80 Mb), the mapping resolution in GWAS is much higher than mouse QTL, so that very limited number of candidate genes are going to be identified. Several large-scale GWAS were conducted for circadian amplitude and for chronotype (such as morningness and eveningness) recently.[86–88] These studies identified a large number of loci, most of which are not canonical clock genes.

These human findings coincide with the previous QTL mapping in mouse crosses[77] and support the notion that the broad variety of circadian behavior observed in humans in phase and in amplitude are the result of polymorphisms in multiple, interacting loci. The number of loci detected in these GWAS was much higher than the mouse study. The differences may reflect the number of samples for GWAS is 2 to 3 log units higher than QTL, or greater genetic diversity in human populations than an experimental cross. Natural variations in human circadian rhythms are subject to complex, polygenic regulation, with allelic variants at large numbers of loci affecting the circadian phenotypes. With the possibility of a hundred or more loci influencing the phenotype, the relative contribution of each genetic locus may be very small.

THE CIRCADIAN TRANSCRIPTOME

As described above, the molecular circadian clock, at its core, is a transcriptional and translational feedback loop, a direct cellular output of which is waves of oscillatory gene expression driven by the rhythmic transcriptional activity of the clock. It has been a central question to understand the program and functional importance of the circadian transcriptome in gene expression profile studies, in which gene expression levels in the SCN and peripheral tissues are accessed at regular time points under entrained (eg, 12-hour light:12-hour dark) or free-running (eg, constant dark) conditions. Early studies have estimated that roughly 30% of the genome is under circadian control.[89–92] This number has been increasing because technical advances in gene expression profiling techniques and larger sample sizes used in subsequent studies. A comprehensive study in mice sampled 12 tissues and found that collectively the expression of 43% of all protein-coding genes showed a circadian rhythmicity.[93] A recent study found an even higher number of genes whose expression was rhythmic in at least 1 tissue of a diurnal primate.[94] These gene expression-profiling studies have revealed a complex circadian transcriptome. First, the circadian transcriptome is highly tissue specific, and only a small fraction of clock-regulated genes is rhythmic across different tissues.[91–95] This tissue specificity appears to be associated with the particular function and metabolic need of the tissue.[91–96] For example, genes rhythmic in the SCN are involved in neuropeptide metabolism and are known for regulating the circadian locomotor activity, whereas genes cycling in the liver are important for nutrient metabolisms and regulation of metabolic intermediates.[91] In addition, the phases (eg, peak time) of the circadian gene expression in a tissue distribute across the entire 24-hour day, as opposed to being restricted to the peak of transcriptional activity of the clock in the tissue, although tissue-specific "rush hours" (times when a large proportion of rhythmic genes have peak transcription) can be observed.[93] Furthermore, even for a gene that is cycling across multiple tissues, the peak of the oscillation can vary by hours in 1 tissue compared with another.[93] The complexity of circadian transcriptomic oscillations across multiple tissues raises an intriguing implication that the circadian transcriptomic program must be under intricate orchestration throughout the body for an overall optimal functional output and health outcome.

Several mechanisms may contribute to this complexity of circadian transcriptome. First, the tissue-specific circadian program in the transcriptome is likely to be associated with tissue-specific configurations of the epigenome, the chemical modifications to the DNA and histone proteins that regulate the binding of transcription factors to regulatory regions of genes and thus the transcriptional activity. Tissue-specific epigenome configurations are critical to establishing cell identity. The epigenome also exhibits clock-regulated circadian oscillations, which correlate with the rhythms in the transcriptome.[97–100] Interestingly, CLOCK shows histone acetyltransferase activity, which modifies chromatin to allow for the accessibility of regulatory elements of genes by transcription factors,[101] a required step for clock-driven circadian transcription activation.[102] Second, in addition to interacting with each other to regulate gene expression, each of the clock proteins also interacts with other transcriptional regulators with distinctive profiles of transcriptional target genes.[103] For example, CLOCK in flies interacts with a range of partner transcription factors and binds to cis-regulatory motifs of genes in a tissue-specific manner, which is associated with the tissue-specific program of circadian transcriptome.[104] Furthermore, by comparing oscillatory patterns of total mRNA to pre-mRNA or nascent mRNA, recent studies suggest that rhythmic transcription activation may only contribute to a portion or even a small portion (eg, 20%–30%) of the rhythms observed in the transcriptome and that post-transcriptional mechanisms are involved.[103,105,106] Consistent with these observations, the transcript levels of hundreds of noncoding regulatory RNAs are also rhythmic.[93,99]

In addition to these cellular mechanisms, the circadian transcriptome is also regulated by systemic signals either directly from the central brain clock in the SCN or indirectly from SCN output rhythms. When the clock machinery was arrested in the liver by tissue-specific inhibition of *Bmal1* expression, 10% of circadian transcriptome remained cycling, suggested a strong contribution from the central clock.[96] Time of feeding, an output rhythm driven by the SCN clock, together with the SCN clock itself, has been shown to drive the rhythms in the hepatic transcriptome in mice.[107,108] Similarly, when mice were sleep deprived at different times of the day so that their sleep debt no longer varied across the circadian cycle, the rhythmic pattern of gene expression in the brain is largely diminished, indicating circadian rhythmic gene expression in the brain is largely dependent on the sleep/wake rhythms.[109] Consistent observations have also been reported in human peripheral blood.[110,111] Finally, body temperature rhythms also reset the phase of the circadian clock in peripheral tissues.[112]

The combination of cellular and systemic mechanisms in shaping the peripheral circadian transcriptomic profiles has important health implications. Under conditions such as jet lag and shift work, the timing signals driven by the SCN clock, behavioral activities, and the local clock are no longer in concert, leading to a state known as the "internal desynchrony." Internal desynchrony is associated with disrupted circadian transcriptome, altered functional outputs, and often disorders. As an example, feeding at a "wrong" time of the day, a condition associated with disrupted metabolic output and deregulation of body weight,[113] creates desynchrony between the transcriptional output of the local clock and systemic signals from the master clock and leads to a reprogrammed circadian transcriptome.[107] Another important health implication of the circadian transcriptome can be drawn from the finding that many genes encoding drug targets or metabolizing enzymes are expressed rhythmically.[93] Thus, the efficacy and toxicity of a drug, particularly one with a short half-life, may be influenced by the time when the drug is taken, a phenomenon that has been reported in circadian pharmacokinetics studies.[114,115]

A challenge of circadian-based drug therapy is the lack of biomarkers of internal timing, which is characteristic of individuals and is highly variable in human populations.[116] Although in principle internal timing can be inferred using transcriptomic and metabolomic data at only 1 time point,[117,118] or with only a few markers in combination with advanced statistical methods,[119] its utility remains to be tested under disease conditions, which typically disrupts circadian transcriptomic patterns, such as seen in the brain of depression patients.[120] In addition, given the complexity of the tissue-specific circadian program, methodologies capable of inferring tissue-specific circadian timing and internal desynchrony are needed. Finally, future studies are needed to demonstrate whether the circadian transcriptome can be used as a disease signature to aid the disease diagnosis, or even as a reference point to treat the disease by restoring the "optimal" cycling pattern. Indeed, these are very challenging tasks at present, particularly given that the circadian transcriptome is also plastic to environmental inputs, such as diet,[121] and are modulated by aging.[122] Nevertheless, with the advances in circadian metabolomics[123] and proteomics,[124–128] we are now beginning to gain an even more detailed understanding of the tissue-specific circadian program and its role in health and disease, building a knowledge base that will eventually enable circadian-based medicine.

SUMMARY: CLOCK GENES ARE EVERYWHERE

The core circadian oscillator can be found in individual cells. The basis for this oscillation in mammals, as in other organisms, lies in rhythmic feedback regulation of transcription of clock genes. The levels of the PER and CRY proteins alter the rate of transcription of their own genes. This alteration is achieved by inhibition of the enhancement of transcription that results from binding of the CLOCK-BMAL1 heterodimer to the E-box element of the promoter region of the Per and Cry genes. Additional interactions between circadian clock proteins may slow the time course of this feedback, achieving the near 24-hour interval: the phosphorylation of PER by CKIε may lead to its degradation, and the association with BMAL1 appears needed for CLOCK to be present in the nucleus. Mutations in core clock genes are involved in the pathogenesis of some familial circadian rhythm sleep-wake disorders. Beyond these core clock genes, rhythmic transcription programs regulate gene expression and gene activity throughout the genome. Finally, it appears that much of the heritability of circadian rhythm traits in mammals stems from polymorphisms in numerous loci beyond the set of core clock genes, with implications for a wide range of neurologic disorders. As computational and molecular techniques mature, future studies are expected to synthesize an understanding of the circadian genetic program at a multiscale level, with important implications for circadian medicine.

ACKNOWLEDGMENTS

Preparation of this article was in part supported by NIH PO1 AG 11412.

REFERENCES

1. Davis FC, Menaker M. Development of the mouse circadian pacemaker: independence from environmental cycles. J Comp Physiol 1981;143(4):527–39.
2. Schwartz WJ, Zimmerman P. Circadian timekeeping in BALB/c and C57BL/6 inbred mouse strains. J Neurosci 1990;10(11):3685–94.
3. Possidente B, Hegmann JP, Carlson L, et al. Pigment mutations associated with altered circadian rhythms in mice. Physiol Behav 1982;28(3):389–92.
4. Ebihara S, Tsuji K, Kondo K. Strain differences of the mouse's free-running circadian rhythm in continuous darkness. Physiol Behav 1978;20(6):795–9.

5. Jiang P, Striz M, Wisor JP, et al. Behavioral and genetic dissection of a mouse model for advanced sleep phase syndrome. Sleep 2011;34(1):39–48.
6. Jiang P, Franklin KM, Duncan MJ, et al. Distinct phase relationships between suprachiasmatic molecular rhythms, cerebral cortex molecular rhythms, and behavioral rhythms in early runner (CAST/EiJ) and nocturnal (C57BL/6J) mice. Sleep 2012;35(10):1385–94.
7. Linkowski P, Van Onderbergen A, Kerkhofs M, et al. Twin study of the 24-h cortisol profile: evidence for genetic control of the human circadian clock. Am J Physiol Endocrinol Metab 1993;264(2):E173–81.
8. Linkowski P. Genetic influences on EEG sleep and the human circadian clock. A twin study. Pharmacopsychiatry 1994;27(1):7–10.
9. Toomey R1, Panizzon MS, Kremen WS, et al. A twin-study of genetic contributions to morningness-eveningness and depression. Chronobiol Int 2015;32(3):303–9.
10. Vink JM1, Groot AS, Kerkhof GA, et al. Genetic analysis of morningness and eveningness. Chronobiol Int 2001;18(5):809–22.
11. Pittendrigh CS. Circadian rhythms and the circadian organization of living systems. Cold Spring Harb Symp Quant Biol 1960;25(0):159–84.
12. Takahashi JS. Molecular neurobiology and genetics of circadian rhythms in mammals. Annu Rev Neurosci 1995;18:531–53.
13. Inouye SIT, Takahashi JS, Wollnik F, et al. Inhibitor of protein synthesis phase shifts a circadian pacemaker in the mammalian SCN. Am J Physiol 1988;255:R1055–8.
14. Watanabe K, Katagai T, Ishida N, et al. Anisomycin induces phase shifts of circadian pacemaker in primary cultures of rat suprachiasmatic nucleus. Brain Res 1995;684(2):179–84.
15. Konopka RJ, Benzer S. Clock mutants of Drosophila melanogaster. Proc Natl Acad Sci U S A 1971;68(9):2112–6.
16. Vitaterna MH, King DP, Chang AM, et al. Mutagenesis and mapping of a mouse gene, Clock, essential for circadian behavior. Science 1994;264(5159):719–25.
17. Dunlap JC. Genetics and molecular analysis of circadian rhythms. Annu Rev Genet 1996;30:579–601.
18. Millar AJ, Carré IA, Strayer CA, et al. Circadian clock mutants in Arabidopsis identified by luciferase imaging. Science 1995;267(5201):1161–3.
19. Kondo T, Tsinoremas NF, Golden SS, et al. Circadian clock mutants of cyanobacteria. Science 1994;266(5188):1233–6.
20. Bargiello TA, Jackson FR, Young MW. Restoration of circadian behavioural rhythms by gene transfer in Drosophila. Nature 1984;312(5996):752–4.
21. Zehring WA, Wheeler DA, Reddy P, et al. P-element transformation with period locus DNA restores rhythmicity to mutant, arrhythmic Drosophila melanogaster. Cell 1984;39(2 Pt 1):369–76.
22. Hardin PE, Hall JC, Rosbash M. Feedback of the Drosophila period gene product on circadian cycling of its messenger RNA levels. Nature 1990;343(6258):536–40.
23. Hardin PE, Hall JC, Rosbash M. Circadian oscillations in period gene mRNA levels are transcriptionally regulated. Proc Natl Acad Sci U S A 1992;89(24):11711–5.
24. Edery I, Zwiebel LJ, Dembinska ME, et al. Temporal phosphorylation of the Drosophila period protein. Proc Natl Acad Sci U S A 1994;91(6):2260–4.
25. Edery I, Rutila JE, Rosbash M. Phase shifting of the circadian clock by induction of the Drosophila period protein. Science 1994;263(5144):237–40.

26. Albrecht U, Sun ZS, Eichele G, et al. A differential response of two putative mammalian circadian regulators, mper1 and mper2, to light. Cell 1997;91(7): 1055–64.

27. Shearman LP, Zylka MJ, Weaver DR, et al. Two period homologs: circadian expression and photic regulation in the suprachiasmatic nuclei. Neuron 1997; 19(6):1261–9.

28. Sun ZS, Albrecht U, Zhuchenko O, et al. RIGUI, a putative mammalian ortholog of the Drosophila period gene. Cell 1997;90(6):1003–11.

29. Tei H, Okamura H, Shigeyoshi Y, et al. Circadian oscillation of a mammalian homologue of the Drosophila period gene. Nature 1997;389(6650):512–6.

30. Zylka MJ, Shearman LP, Weaver DR, et al. Three period homologs in mammals: differential light responses in the suprachiasmatic circadian clock and oscillating transcripts outside of brain. Neuron 1998;20(6):1103–10.

31. King DP, Vitaterna MH, Chang AM, et al. The mouse Clock mutation behaves as an antimorph and maps within the W19H deletion, distal of Kit. Genetics 1997; 146(3):1049–60.

32. Antoch MP, Song EJ, Chang AM, et al. Functional identification of the mouse circadian Clock gene by transgenic BAC rescue. Cell 1997;89(4):655–67.

33. King DP, Zhao Y, Sangoram AM, et al. Positional cloning of the mouse circadian clock gene. Cell 1997;89(4):641–53.

34. Gekakis N, Staknis D, Nguyen HB, et al. Role of the CLOCK protein in the mammalian circadian mechanism. Science 1998;280(5369):1564–9.

35. Kondratov RV, Chernov MV, Kondratova AA, et al. BMAL1-dependent circadian oscillation of nuclear CLOCK: posttranslational events induced by dimerization of transcriptional activators of the mammalian clock system. Genes Dev 2003; 17(15):1921–32.

36. Hao H, Allen DL, Hardin PE. A circadian enhancer mediates PER-dependent mRNA cycling in Drosophila melanogaster. Mol Cell Biol 1997;17(7):3687–93.

37. Bunger MK, Wilsbacher LD, Moran SM, et al. Mop3 is an essential component of the master circadian pacemaker in mammals. Cell 2000;103(7):1009–17.

38. Shearman L, Weaver D. Photic induction of Period gene expression is reduced in Clock mutant mice. Neuroreport 1999;10(3):613–8.

39. Bae K, Jin X, Maywood ES, et al. Differential functions of mPer1, mPer2, and mPer3 in the SCN circadian clock. Neuron 2001;30(2):525–36.

40. Zheng B, Albrecht U, Kaasik K, et al. Nonredundant roles of the mPer1 and mPer2 genes in the mammalian circadian clock. Cell 2001;105(5):683–94.

41. Miyamoto Y, Sancar A. Vitamin B2-based blue-light photoreceptors in the retinohypothalamic tract as the photoactive pigments for setting the circadian clock in mammals. Proc Natl Acad Sci U S A 1998;95(11):6097–102.

42. Thresher RJ, Vitaterna MH, Miyamoto Y, et al. Role of mouse cryptochrome blue-light photoreceptor in circadian photoresponses. Science 1998;282(5393): 1490–4.

43. Vitaterna MH, Selby CP, Todo T, et al. Differential regulation of mammalian period genes and circadian rhythmicity by cryptochromes 1 and 2. Proc Natl Acad Sci U S A 1999;96(21):12114–9.

44. van der Horst GT, Muijtjens M, Kobayashi K, et al. Mammalian Cry1 and Cry2 are essential for maintenance of circadian rhythms. Nature 1999;398(6728): 627–30.

45. Okamura H, Miyake S, Sumi Y, et al. Photic induction of mPer1 and mPer2 in cry-deficient mice lacking a biological clock. Science 1999;286(5449):2531–4.

46. Kume K, Zylka MJ, Sriram S, et al. mCRY1 and mCRY2 are essential components of the negative limb of the circadian clock feedback loop. Cell 1999; 98(2):193–205.

47. Ralph MR, Menaker M. A mutation of the circadian system in golden hamsters. Science 1988;241(4870):1225–7.

48. Shimomura K, Menaker M. Light-induced phase shifts in tau mutant hamsters. J Biol Rhythms 1994;9(2):97–110.

49. Lowrey PL, Shimomura K, Antoch MP, et al. Positional syntenic cloning and functional characterization of the mammalian circadian mutation tau. Science 2000; 288(5465):483–92.

50. Etchegaray JP, Yu EA, Indic P, et al. Casein kinase 1 delta (CK1delta) regulates period length of the mouse suprachiasmatic circadian clock in vitro. PLoS One 2010;5(4):e10303.

51. Xu Y, Padiath QS, Shapiro RE, et al. Functional consequences of a CKIdelta mutation causing familial advanced sleep phase syndrome. Nature 2005; 434(7033):640–4.

52. Isojima Y, Nakajima M, Ukai H, et al. CKIepsilon/delta-dependent phosphorylation is a temperature-insensitive, period-determining process in the mammalian circadian clock. Proc Natl Acad Sci U S A 2009;106(37):15744–9.

53. Lee H, Chen R, Lee Y, et al. Essential roles of CKIdelta and CKIepsilon in the mammalian circadian clock. Proc Natl Acad Sci U S A 2009;106(50):21359–64.

54. Preitner N, Damiola F, Lopez-Molina L, et al. The orphan nuclear receptor REV-ERBalpha controls circadian transcription within the positive limb of the mammalian circadian oscillator. Cell 2002;110(2):251–60.

55. Asher G, Gatfield D, Stratmann M, et al. SIRT1 regulates Circadian clock gene expression through PER2 deacetylation. Cell 2008;134(2):317–28.

56. Nakahata Y, Kaluzova M, Grimaldi B, et al. The NAD+-dependent deacetylase SIRT1 modulates CLOCK-mediated chromatin remodeling and circadian control. Cell 2008;134(2):329–40.

57. Nakahata Y, Sahar S, Astarita G, et al. Circadian control of the NAD+ salvage pathway by CLOCK-SIRT1. Science 2009;324(5927):654–7.

58. Ramsey KM, Yoshino J, Brace CS, et al. Circadian clock feedback cycle through NAMPT-mediated NAD+ biosynthesis. Science 2009;324(5927):651–4.

59. Etchegaray JP, Lee C, Wade PA, et al. Rhythmic histone acetylation underlies transcription in the mammalian circadian clock. Nature 2003;421(6919):177–82.

60. Liu AC, Tran HG, Zhang EE, et al. Redundant function of REV-ERBα and β and non-essential role for bmal1 cycling in transcriptional regulation of intracellular circadian rhythms. PLoS Genet 2008;4(2):e1000023.

61. Siepka SM, Yoo SH, Park J, et al. Circadian mutant overtime reveals f-box protein fbxl3 regulation of cryptochrome and period gene expression. Cell 2007; 129(5):1011–23.

62. Dardente H, Mendoza J, Fustin JM, et al. Implication of the F-Box Protein FBXL21 in circadian pacemaker function in mammals. PLoS One 2008;3(10): e3530.

63. Hirano A, Yumimoto K, Tsunematsu R, et al. FBXL21 regulates oscillation of the circadian clock through ubiquitination and stabilization of cryptochromes. Cell 2013;152(5):1106–18.

64. Yoo SH, Mohawk JA, Siepka SM, et al. Competing E3 ubiquitin ligases govern circadian periodicity by degradation of CRY in nucleus and cytoplasm. Cell 2013;152(5):1091–105.

65. Reick M, Garcia JA, Dudley C, et al. NPAS2: an analog of clock operative in the mammalian forebrain. Science 2001;293(5529):506–9.
66. DeBruyne JP, Noton E, Lambert CM, et al. A clock shock: mouse CLOCK is not required for circadian oscillator function. Neuron 2006;50(3):465–77.
67. DeBruyne JP, Weaver DR, Reppert SM. CLOCK and NPAS2 have overlapping roles in the suprachiasmatic circadian clock. Nat Neurosci 2007;10(5):543–5.
68. Honma S, Kawamoto T, Takagi Y, et al. Dec1 and Dec2 are regulators of the mammalian molecular clock. Nature 2002;419(6909):841–4.
69. Sato F, Kawamoto T, Fujimoto K, et al. Functional analysis of the basic helix-loop-helix transcription factor DEC1 in circadian regulation. Interaction with BMAL1. Eur J Biochem 2004;271(22):4409–19.
70. Li Y, Song X, Ma Y, et al. DNA binding, but not interaction with Bmal1, is responsible for DEC1-mediated transcription regulation of the circadian gene mPer1. Biochem J 2004;382(3):895–904.
71. He Y, Jones CR, Fujiki N, et al. The transcriptional repressor DEC2 regulates sleep length in mammals. Science 2009;325(5942):866–70.
72. Patke A, Murphy PJ, Onat OE, et al. Mutation of the human circadian clock gene CRY1 in familial delayed sleep phase disorder. Cell 2017;169(2):203–15.
73. Von Schantz M. Natural variation in Human Clocks. Adv Genet 2017;99:73–96.
74. Toh KL, Jones CR, He Y, et al. An hPer2 phosphorylation site mutation in familial advanced sleep phase syndrome. Science 2001;291(5506):1040–3.
75. Hirano A, Shi G, Jones CR, et al. A Cryptochrome 2 mutation yields advanced sleep phase in humans. Elife 2016;5 [pii:e16695].
76. Shanware NP, Hutchinson JA, Kim SH, et al. Casein kinase 1-dependent phosphorylation of familial advanced sleep phase syndrome-associated residues controls PERIOD 2 stability. J Biol Chem 2011;286(14):12766–74.
77. Shimomura K, Low-Zeddies SS, King DP, et al. Genome-wide epistatic interaction analysis reveals complex genetic determinants of circadian behavior in mice. Genome Res 2001;11(6):959–80.
78. Shimomura K, Lowrey PL, Vitaterna MH, et al. Genetic suppression of the circadian Clock mutation by the melatonin biosynthesis pathway. Proc Natl Acad Sci U S A 2010;107(18):8399–403.
79. Roseboom PH, Namboodiri MA, Zimonjic DB, et al. Natural melatonin 'knockdown' in C57BL/6J mice: rare mechanism truncates serotonin N-acetyltransferase. Brain Res Mol Brain Res 1998;63(1):189–97.
80. Kasahara T, Abe K, Mekada K, et al. Genetic variation of melatonin productivity in laboratory mice under domestication. Proc Natl Acad Sci U S A 2010;107(14):6412–7.
81. Turek FW, Joshu C, Kohsaka A, et al. Obesity and metabolic syndrome in circadian Clock mutant mice. Science 2005;308(5724):1043–5.
82. Bouatia-Naji N, Bonnefond A, Cavalcanti-Proenca C, et al. A variant near MTNR1B is associated with increased fasting plasma glucose levels and type 2 diabetes risk. Nat Genet 2009;41(1):89–94.
83. Lyssenko V, Nagorny CL, Erdos MR, et al. Common variant in MTNR1B associated with increased risk of type 2 diabetes and impaired early insulin secretion. Nat Genet 2009;41(1):82–8.
84. Prokopenko I, Langenberg C, Florez JC, et al. Variants in MTNR1B influence fasting glucose levels. Nat Genet 2009;41(1):77–81.
85. Shimomura K, Kumar V, Koike N, et al. Usf1, a suppressor of the circadian Clock mutant, reveals the nature of the DNA-binding of the CLOCK:BMAL1 complex in mice. Elife 2013;2:e00426.

86. Ferguson A, Lyall LM, Ward J, et al. Genome-wide association study of circadian rhythmicity in 71,500 uk biobank participants and polygenic association with mood instability. EBioMedicine 2018;35:279–87.

87. Dashti HS, Jones SE, Wood AR, et al. Genome-wide association study identifies genetic loci for self-reported habitual sleep duration supported by accelerometer-derived estimates. Nat Commun 2019;10(1):1100.

88. Jones SE, Lane JM, Wood AR, et al. Genome-wide association analyses of chronotype in 697,828 individuals provides insights into circadian rhythms. Nat Commun 2019;10(1):343.

89. Akhtar RA, Reddy AB, Maywood ES, et al. Circadian cycling of the mouse liver transcriptome, as revealed by cDNA microarray, is driven by the suprachiasmatic nucleus. Curr Biol 2002;12(7):540–50.

90. Duffield GE, Best JD, Meurers BH, et al. Circadian programs of transcriptional activation, signaling, and protein turnover revealed by microarray analysis of mammalian cells. Curr Biol 2002;12(7):551–7.

91. Panda S, Antoch MP, Miller BH, et al. Coordinated transcription of key pathways in the mouse by the circadian clock. Cell 2002;109(3):307–20.

92. Storch K-F, Lipan O, Leykin I, et al. Extensive and divergent circadian gene expression in liver and heart. Nature 2002;417(6884):78–83.

93. Zhang R, Lahens NF, Ballance HI, et al. A circadian gene expression atlas in mammals: implications for biology and medicine. Proc Natl Acad Sci U S A 2014;111(45):16219–24.

94. Mure LS, Le HD, Benegiamo G, et al. Diurnal transcriptome atlas of a primate across major neural and peripheral tissues. Science 2018;359(6381):eaao0318.

95. Miller BH, McDearmon EL, Panda S, et al. Circadian and CLOCK-controlled regulation of the mouse transcriptome and cell proliferation. Proc Natl Acad Sci U S A 2007;104(9):3342–7.

96. Kornmann B, Schaad O, Bujard H, et al. System-driven and oscillator-dependent circadian transcription in mice with a conditionally active liver clock. PLoS Biol 2007;5(2):e34.

97. Le Martelot G, Canella D, Symul L, et al. Genome-wide RNA polymerase II profiles and RNA accumulation reveal kinetics of transcription and associated epigenetic changes during diurnal cycles. PLoS Biol 2012;10(11):e1001442.

98. Rey G, Cesbron F, Rougemont J, et al. Genome-wide and phase-specific DNA-binding rhythms of BMAL1 control circadian output functions in mouse liver. PLoS Biol 2011;9(2):e1000595.

99. Vollmers C, Schmitz Robert J, Nathanson J, et al. Circadian oscillations of protein-coding and regulatory RNAs in a highly dynamic mammalian liver epigenome. Cell Metab 2012;16(6):833–45.

100. Papazyan R, Zhang Y, Lazar MA. Genetic and epigenomic mechanisms of mammalian circadian transcription. Nat Struct Mol Biol 2016;23:1045.

101. Menet JS, Pescatore S, Rosbash M. CLOCK:BMAL1 is a pioneer-like transcription factor. Genes Dev 2014;28(1):8–13.

102. Doi M, Hirayama J, Sassone-Corsi P. Circadian regulator CLOCK is a histone acetyltransferase. Cell 2006;125(3):497–508.

103. Koike N, Yoo S-H, Huang H-C, et al. Transcriptional architecture and chromatin landscape of the core circadian clock in mammals. Science 2012;338(6105):349–54.

104. Meireles-Filho Antonio CA, Bardet Anaïs F, Yáñez-Cuna JO, et al. cis-Regulatory requirements for tissue-specific programs of the circadian clock. Curr Biol 2014;24(1):1–10.

105. Menet JS, Rodriguez J, Abruzzi KC, et al. Nascent-Seq reveals novel features of mouse circadian transcriptional regulation. Elife 2012;1:e00011.
106. Rodriguez J, Tang C-HA, Khodor YL, et al. Nascent-Seq analysis of Drosophila cycling gene expression. Proc Natl Acad Sci U S A 2013;110(4):E275–84.
107. Vollmers C, Gill S, DiTacchio L, et al. Time of feeding and the intrinsic circadian clock drive rhythms in hepatic gene expression. Proc Natl Acad Sci U S A 2009; 106(50):21453–8.
108. Greenwell BJ, Trott AJ, Beytebiere JR, et al. Rhythmic food intake drives rhythmic gene expression more potently than the hepatic circadian clock in mice. Cell Rep 2019;27(3):649–57.e5.
109. Maret S, Dorsaz S, Gurcel L, et al. Homer1a is a core brain molecular correlate of sleep loss. Proc Natl Acad Sci U S A 2007;104(50):20090–5.
110. Möller-Levet CS, Archer SN, Bucca G, et al. Effects of insufficient sleep on circadian rhythmicity and expression amplitude of the human blood transcriptome. Proc Natl Acad Sci U S A 2013;110(12):E1132–41.
111. Archer SN, Laing EE, Möller-Levet CS, et al. Mistimed sleep disrupts circadian regulation of the human transcriptome. Proc Natl Acad Sci U S A 2014;111(6): E682–91.
112. Buhr ED, Yoo SH, Takahashi JS. Temperature as a universal resetting cue for mammalian circadian oscillators. Science 2010;330(6002):379–85.
113. Jiang P, Turek FW. The endogenous circadian clock programs animals to eat at certain times of the 24-hour day: what if we ignore the clock? Physiol Behav 2018;193(Pt B):211–7.
114. Griffett K, Burris TP. The mammalian clock and chronopharmacology. Bioorg Med Chem Lett 2013;23(7):1929–34.
115. Dallmann R, Okyar A, Lévi F. Dosing-time makes the poison: circadian regulation and pharmacotherapy. Trends Mol Med 2016;22(5):430–45.
116. Fischer D, Lombardi DA, Marucci-Wellman H, et al. Chronotypes in the US—influence of age and sex. PLoS One 2017;12(6):e0178782.
117. Kasukawa T, Sugimoto M, Hida A, et al. Human blood metabolite timetable indicates internal body time. Proc Natl Acad Sci U S A 2012;109(37):15036–41.
118. Ueda HR, Chen W, Minami Y, et al. Molecular-timetable methods for detection of body time and rhythm disorders from single-time-point genome-wide expression profiles. Proc Natl Acad Sci U S A 2004;101(31):11227–32.
119. Braun R, Kath WL, Iwanaszko M, et al. Universal method for robust detection of circadian state from gene expression. Proc Natl Acad Sci U S A 2018;115(39): E9247–56.
120. Li JZ, Bunney BG, Meng F, et al. Circadian patterns of gene expression in the human brain and disruption in major depressive disorder. Proc Natl Acad Sci U S A 2013;110(24):9950–5.
121. Eckel-Mahan Kristin L, Patel Vishal R, de Mateo S, et al. Reprogramming of the circadian clock by nutritional challenge. Cell 2013;155(7):1464–78.
122. Sato S, Solanas G, Peixoto FO, et al. Circadian reprogramming in the liver identifies metabolic pathways of aging. Cell 2017;170(4):664–77.e11.
123. Dyar KA, Eckel-Mahan KL. Circadian metabolomics in time and space. Front Neurosci 2017;11:369.
124. Hurley JM, Jankowski MS, De Los Santos H, et al. Circadian proteomic analysis uncovers mechanisms of post-transcriptional regulation in metabolic pathways. Cell Syst 2018;7(6):613–26.e5.

125. Schenk S, Bannister SC, Sedlazeck FJ, et al. Combined transcriptome and proteome profiling reveals specific molecular brain signatures for sex, maturation and circalunar clock phase. Elife 2019;8 [pii:e41556].
126. Wang Y, Song L, Liu M, et al. A proteomics landscape of circadian clock in mouse liver. Nat Commun 2018;9(1):1553.
127. Wang J, Mauvoisin D, Martin E, et al. Nuclear proteomics uncovers diurnal regulatory landscapes in mouse liver. Cell Metab 2017;25(1):102–17.
128. Robles MS, Humphrey SJ, Mann M. Phosphorylation is a central mechanism for circadian control of metabolism and physiology. Cell Metab 2017;25(1):118–27.

Assessment of Circadian Rhythms

Kathryn J. Reid, PhD

KEYWORDS

- Dim light melatonin onset • Core body temperature • Circadian rhythms
- Rest-activity cycles • Circadian rhythm sleep-wake disorders

KEY POINTS

- Assessment of circadian rhythms is likely to benefit the diagnosis, treatment, and long-term management of those with circadian rhythm sleep-wake disorders.
- The dim light melatonin onset is the current gold-standard marker of circadian phase.
- The degree of circadian disruption may be a marker of severity of the disorder and direct the selection of treatment strategies.
- Development of new comprehensive tools to assess circadian rhythms across a variety of domains such as expression of molecular clocks may lead to better management and targeted treatment of circadian rhythm sleep-wake disorders.

INTRODUCTION

The focus of this article is to review several commonly used methods for the assessment of circadian rhythms as it relates to circadian rhythm sleep-wake disorders (CRSWDs).[1] It also touches on recent research on the development of new biomarkers of the circadian system in humans. The goal of this article is not to provide specific details of the methods to assess circadian rhythms; rather, it is to review the key factors to consider when selecting a method and when collecting and interpreting the data from these measures. Reference to works that do provide more detail on the methods themselves is provided within each section.

To set the stage, the reader must first have an understanding of the circadian system, the factors that influence (or mask) the outputs (or markers) of the circadian system, and the terminology used to describe the circadian system. There are numerous output rhythms of the circadian system that can be assessed to determine the phase, amplitude, and period of the circadian system. A graphic representation of these circadian

Disclosure Statement: The author has nothing to disclose.
Department of Neurology, Center for Circadian and Sleep Medicine, Northwestern University Feinberg School of Medicine, 710 North Lakeshore Drive, Abbott Hall Room 522, Chicago, IL 60611, USA
E-mail address: k-reid@northwestern.edu

Neurol Clin 37 (2019) 505–526
https://doi.org/10.1016/j.ncl.2019.05.001
0733-8619/19/© 2019 Elsevier Inc. All rights reserved.

neurologic.theclinics.com

concepts is provided in **Fig. 1**; the difference in the level between peak and trough values is the amplitude of the rhythm. The timing of a reference point in the cycle (eg, the peak) relative to a fixed event (eg, beginning of the night phase) is the phase. The time interval between phase reference points (eg, 2 peaks) is called the period.[2]

Assessment of circadian rhythms in clinical practice can serve several functions; the most important of these is the ability to determine the extent of circadian disruption or the misalignment of circadian rhythms with the external environment. Another practical reason is to precisely time circadian-based treatments such as bright light exposure and exogenous melatonin administration. The timing of these treatments relative to the internal circadian clock will determine whether they result in phase advances or phase delays, and this response can be expressed graphically as a phase response curve.[3–7] A simplified example is that light exposure before the core body temperature (CBT) minimum results in phase delays of the circadian clock and light after the core temperature minimum results in phase advances.[7] Mistiming of circadian-based treatments such as light and melatonin may worsen circadian disturbance and exacerbate other symptoms. Currently the most common way that clinicians determine the appropriate time to administer these treatments is by setting a time relative to either sleep start or end times. This strategy makes certain assumptions about the phase relationship between various circadian rhythm outputs such as sleep, melatonin onset, and CBT minimum. Another reason to assess circadian rhythms is to better understand the pathophysiology of circadian rhythm disorders. There is recent evidence to suggest that not all individuals who meet the current clinical criteria for delayed sleep-wake phase disorder have a delayed circadian phase of melatonin, even though their sleep-wake cycle is delayed.[8,9] Because many circadian-based treatments are currently scheduled relative to sleep timing, the lack of a delayed melatonin rhythm in some patients with delayed sleep-wake phase disorder could make appropriate timing of circadian-based treatments difficult and could explain why there have been mixed results in the literature in studies using circadian-based treatment in this population.[10]

Finally, the need to assess the timing, amplitude, and alignment of the various outputs of the circadian system is supported by growing evidence to suggest that

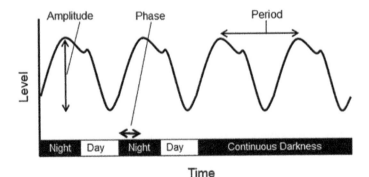

Fig. 1. Parameters of circadian rhythms. A representative circadian rhythm is depicted in which the level of a particular measure (eg, blood hormone levels and activity levels) varies according to time. The difference in the level between peak and trough values is the *amplitude* of the rhythm. The timing of a reference point in the cycle (eg, the peak) relative to a fixed event (eg, beginning of the night phase) is the *phase*. The time interval between phase reference points (eg, 2 peaks) is called the *period*. The rhythm shown persists even in continuous darkness (ie, free running). (*From* Vitaterna MH, Takahashi JS, Turek FW. Overview of circadian rhythms. Alcohol Res Health 2001;25:85-93; with permission)

misalignment of circadian rhythms in central and peripheral tissues can lead not only to poor sleep but also to poor physical and mental health outcomes.[11]

CIRCADIAN RHYTHMS

The sleep-wake cycle is perhaps the most prominent circadian rhythm in humans. Circadian rhythms, which are present in virtually all physiologic and behavioral functions, are generated by a circadian pacemaker located in the suprachiasmatic nuclei (SCN) of the anterior hypothalamus.[12–15] The circadian timing system is conceptualized as 3 distinct components: a circadian oscillator with a rhythm approximating 24 hours, input pathways for light and other stimuli that synchronize the pacemaker to the environmental light/dark cycle (zeitgebers), and output rhythms that are regulated by the pacemaker. Circadian rhythms are intrinsic to the organism, and in the absence of synchronizing stimuli, they will continue with a period of approximately 24 hours.[16] Circadian rhythms are synchronized to the environmental light/dark and social/activity cycles by daily adjustments in the timing (the phase) of the rhythm[16]; this process is called entrainment.

In humans, light is the most effective synchronizing agent for the clock. Photic information reaches the circadian system via a direct pathway, the retinohypothalamic tract,[17] and an indirect pathway via the intergeniculate leaflet.[18] It is now recognized that the primary circadian photoreceptors are the intrinsically photosensitive melanopsin-containing retinal ganglion cells.[19,20] Furthermore, both light-induced phase shifts and melatonin suppression are most sensitive to short-wavelength light at approximately 460 nm.[21,22] In addition to light exposure, exogenous melatonin administration and physical activity have also been shown to induce changes in the phase of circadian rhythms.[23,24]

Regulation of the human sleep-wake cycle is generated by a complex interaction of endogenous circadian (process C) and homeostatic (process S) processes as well as environmental factors.[25,26] Process C is driven by the circadian clock that promotes wakefulness during the day and facilitates the consolidation of sleep during the night.[27–31] Maximum alertness occurs in the early evening hours when the drive for sleep is also highest.[32–36] The amount and depth of sleep is instead determined by the sleep homeostatic process. The homeostatic process of sleep accumulates as a function of prior wakefulness; currently sleep is the only known way to reduce this homeostatic drive after extended wakefulness.[25,37,38] Therefore, proper alignment between circadian timing of sleep-wake and other behaviors such as feeding are essential for optimal sleep, waking function, and health.[11,39–45]

COMMON MEASURES USED TO ASSESS CIRCADIAN RHYTHMS

Circadian rhythms can be observed in almost all physiologic functions, but in humans there have been 3 main outputs used to assess circadian rhythms to date: melatonin levels, CBT, and rest-activity cycles. Given limited availability of some of these objective measures in the clinical setting, other tools such as sleep diaries and chronotype questionnaires can be used to aid clinical diagnosis of CRSWDs.

In the clinical setting, most markers of circadian timing are collected in the field/home while patients are going about their usual daily activities. However, given the masking effects of light, activity (including sleep-wake), and feeding on some of these measures, the use of specialized protocols within the laboratory setting specifically designed to minimize the influence of these factors is often preferred to obtain an accurate assessment of the underlying circadian timing (ie, constant routine, forced desynchrony[33,46–48]). The down side to a laboratory-based approach is that people do not "live" in a laboratory, and understanding the interaction between circadian, environmental, and behavioral factors may be important for diagnosis and management in clinical care. Given this, some key factors to consider when instructing patients on the collection of the measure and in the interpretation of the data are provided for each circadian marker discussed.

Although the measurement of the dim light melatonin onset (DLMO) is encouraged in the diagnostic criteria for some CRSWDs,[1] there are no specific guidelines for which technique to determine DLMO is the best for clinical purposes, and there are benefits and disadvantages to each method. In general terms, when selecting a method to determine circadian rhythms, consideration should be given to what you are trying to measure; what the population is; whether the samples will be collected at home or in the laboratory; the level of invasiveness; the sampling period; and frequency to be assessed whether it be a single evening, a full 24-hour period, or even assessment over multiple days. Cost is also a major consideration; many of these tests cannot currently be claimed with medical insurance and are an out-of-pocket cost, which in some cases limits these tests to those that can afford it.

SLEEP LOG/DIARY

Keeping a daily sleep log/diary for 14 days (minimum 7 days) on both work/school days and free days is part of the Internal Classification of Sleep Disorders diagnostic criteria for the following CRSWDs: delayed sleep-wake phase disorder, advanced sleep-wake phase disorder, non-24-hour sleep-wake rhythm disorder (minimum 14 days), irregular sleep-wake rhythm disorder, and shift work disorder.[1] Sleep logs allow the clinician to characterize the pattern of sleep-wake. Sleep logs should include information about the day of the week, whether it is a work/school or free day, when the person went to bed, when they fell asleep, when they woke up, and when they got out of bed. It is also useful if the sleep log contains information about other behaviors such as when the patient took medications, when they consumed caffeine or alcohol, and when they napped or exercised. The American Academy of Sleep Medicine has a sample 2-week sleep diary available on the web.[49] Another useful piece of information that can be captured on the sleep log is the start and end of electronics use each day. Electronic devices emit light, and depending on the activities they are being used for, they may be alerting (video games, movies) which could exacerbate sleep-wake and circadian disturbance in those with sleep disorders.

CIRCADIAN CHRONOTYPE

A tool frequently used as a proxy of the timing of the circadian system is circadian preference or chronotype assessed via questionnaires.[50,51] Circadian chronotype is typically defined by a person's preferred time to conduct daily activities[50] and or the timing of sleep.[51,52] The most commonly used questionnaires are the Morningness-Eveningness Questionnaire,[50] the Munich Chronotype Questionnaire (MCTQ), and the Munich Chronotype Questionnaire for Shift-Workers (MCTQShift).[51,53] Although these questionnaires align reasonably well in healthy controls with other measures of the circadian system such a CBT and melatonin levels,[54–58] in patient populations these relationships are less clear.

These questionnaires do not measure circadian rhythms per se, but they can still be useful tools to identify extreme early or late types and to characterize concepts such as "social jetlag."[59] The International Classification of Sleep Disorders criteria now suggest that standardized chronotype questionnaires can be useful tools to assess chronotype in those with advanced or delayed sleep-wake phase disorder.[1] So even though an extreme morning (lark) or evening (owl) type preference on the Morningness-Eveningness Questionnaire does not indicate a CRSWD, those with delayed sleep-wake phase disorder tend to be extreme evening types[60,61] and those with advanced sleep-wake phase disorder tend to be extreme morning types.[62]

One of the most prominent features of the difference between morning/evening types is that they exhibit different timing to patterns of sleep-wake.[50,63,64] Morning types have also been reported to be less flexible particularly in their rising times, than evening types.[65] There is also evidence that there are alterations in the dissipation and buildup of homeostatic sleep drive in those with extreme circadian preference but a normal circadian phase (ie, intermediate time of DLMO), which is not present in those with both an extreme circadian preference and extreme circadian phase (ie, early or late DLMO).[66,67]

The MCTQ is considerably newer than the Morningness-Eveningness Questionnaire and uses a different approach to determine circadian chronotype. Although the Morningness-Eveningness Questionnaire includes questions related to an individual's preference of the timing of various daily activities including sleep,[50] the MCTQ estimates chronotype based on the midpoint between sleep onset and offset on work-free days, corrected for "oversleep" due to the sleep debt that individuals accumulate over the workweek.[51] Chronotype as measured by the MCTQ is based on the assumption that sleep timing on work-free days is highly influenced by the circadian clock. The discrepancy between work and free days, between social and biological time, can be described as "social jetlag."[59] The MCTQ has been taken by hundreds of thousands of people online and "social jetlag" has been shown to be associated with age, body mass index, and other poor health behaviors and outcomes.[51,59,68,69]

REST-ACTIVITY RHYTHMS

Rest-activity rhythms are one of the most prominent outputs of the circadian system. Although the control of sleep timing and quality is a combination of the interaction between both homeostatic and circadian processes, it can be significantly influenced by behavior. So although rest-activity rhythms are commonly used to assess circadian function in both animals and humans, they are not purely a function of the circadian clock. Wrist activity monitoring in humans is commonly used to assess the timing of rest-activity cycles as a proxy of circadian timing. Detailed recommendations for how and when to use actigraphy in the clinical setting are available from various sources.[70–73] In fact, assessing the pattern of sleep-wake over 14 days (minimum 7 days) using sleep diary or wrist actigraphy with a sleep diary is part of the diagnostic criteria for the following CRSWDs: delayed sleep-wake phase disorder, advanced sleep-wake phase disorder, non-24-hour sleep-wake rhythm disorder (minimum 14 days), irregular sleep-wake rhythm disorder, and shift work disorder.[1] An example of why this can be helpful is depicted in the actogram of wrist activity monitoring from a patient with non-24-hour sleep-wake rhythm disorder provided in **Fig. 2**. Of note in this example is that the rest period moves about an hour later each day, a key feature of non-24-hour sleep-wake disorder. It has also been shown that the circadian rhythm of melatonin and CBT will also progressively delay along with the rest-activity cycles in these patients.[74]

Several measures can be determined using information from rest-activity cycles that are thought to reflect the strength and timing of the circadian system. The measures derived from the rest-activity cycles have been shown to be associated with morbidity and mortality, changes in response to an intervention, and even neurodegenerative disorders.[75–78] Estimates of sleep-wake timing are just one of the

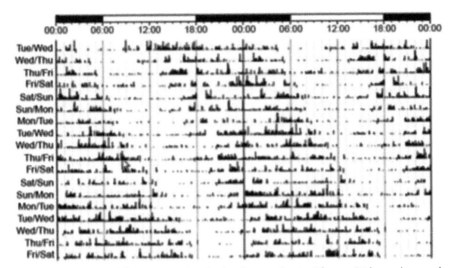

Fig. 2. An example of the rest-activity rhythm in a patient with non-24-hour sleep-wake phase disorder recorded with wrist activity monitoring. In this figure activity level (dark tick marks) is double plotted, which means that each line includes 2 days between mid-night to mid-night and that part of the second day is plotted on the line below. The rest-activity rhythm in those with non-24-hour sleep-wake phase disorder typically progressively delays each day so that at certain times the rest period occurs during the daytime. (*From* Reid KJ, Zee PC. Circadian Rhythm Sleep Disorders. In: Kryger M, ed. Atlas of Clinical Sleep Medicine. 2nd ed: Saunder, Elsevier, 2013; with permission.)

"circadian rhythm" variables that can be extracted from activity records. Most commercially available wrist-worn activity monitors use propriety algorithms to estimate sleep-wake, and from these you are able to ascertain sleep onset, offset, and sleep midpoint (clock time that represents the midpoint between sleep onset and end of the sleep offset[39,79]). Later sleep midpoint (typically after 5 AM) in particular has been shown to be associated with numerous poor cardiometabolic health outcomes.[39,79] An example of wrist actigraphy from a healthy older individual is provided in **Fig. 3**; the average bedtime and wake time for this individual are 11:40 PM and 08:00 AM respectively, total sleep time is about 7.5 hours.

Another feature that is available in some actigraphy devices (see **Figs. 3** and **8**) is the ability to measure light levels. Although measuring light levels at the wrist has its limitations and may not accurately reflect light exposure at the eye, there is evidence to suggest that light levels determined with actigraphy are associated with sleep quality, mood, and health-related outcomes.[80–82] By monitoring when patients are exposed to relatively bright light, clinicians are able to guide patients on how to modify behaviors to reduce light exposure at the wrong circadian time, as this may be perpetuating or exacerbating their circadian disturbance. Alternatively, it can also provide information about when to increase light levels to enhance phase shifting or circadian entrainment.[61,83,84]

Other measures of circadian activity rhythms (CAR) have been developed and applied to various populations. CAR methods have used traditional cosine models[85] and more frequently now newer expanded versions of these traditional cosine models are used to map the CAR to activity data.[75–77,86–88] CAR measures include amplitude, a measure of the strength of the activity rhythm; mesor, the mean level of activity; and the acrophase or time of day of peak activity. Another of these measures is the pseudo

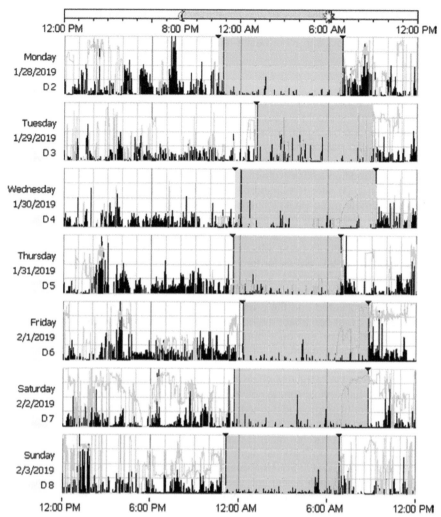

Fig. 3. An example of the rest-activity rhythm from a healthy older adult recorded with wrist activity monitoring. Each row is a 24-hour day from 12 PM to 12 PM the next day. Activity levels are indicated in black and light levels in yellow. The light blue shaded area indicates the sleep period. The small blue triangles at the beginning and end of the light blue shaded sleep period are markers selected by the individual to indicate when they went to bed and when they woke up. The individual has a stable nocturnal sleep-wake period and woke up several times during the night (an example of this can be seen on day 3 as the increase in activity and light within the sleep period).

F-statistic that represents a measure of the robustness of CAR, with higher pseudo-F values indicating stronger rhythms.[89]

There are also other nonparametric variables that can be determined from wrist activity monitoring that are believed to reflect rhythmic behavior.[90,91] These variables include interdaily stability, intradaily variability, and relative amplitude of activity values, the start times and average activity of M10 (ie, 10 hours with maximal activity) and L5 (ie, 5 hours with least activity). The code to calculate these measures has been published by Blume and colleagues.[92] These measures can be improved with circadian-based interventions and have been associated with dementia, diabetes, blood pressure, mood, and other health-related measures.[11,90,93]

MELATONIN

Melatonin is an endogenous hormone synthesized and released by the pineal gland, and the onset of melatonin production is commonly used as a marker of the timing of the endogenous circadian system.[94–96] Melatonin secretion is controlled by way of a multisynaptic neural pathway consisting of sympathetic innervations, through the SCN, preganglionic neurons, and postganglionic fibers from the superior cervical ganglion.[95] In addition to being used as a marker of the circadian system, melatonin has the ability to (1) alter the timing of circadian rhythms (phase shifting[3,97,98]) and (2) help to promote sleep via its influence on the SCN, as melatonin inhibits the firing rate of SCN neurons creating a sleep permissive state.[99,100]

Melatonin can be detected in plasma and saliva and its major metabolite 6-sulpha-toxymelatonin (aMT6s) in urine. Melatonin levels are most commonly measured in plasma or saliva, as this allows for frequent sampling ($\sim$ every 30 minutes) for more precise determination of phase. Each of these approaches comes with its own specific sampling methods and considerations, including the environment in which the sample will be collected and the presence of certain medications[101–103] and health conditions[104,105] that can affect the accuracy of the melatonin levels detected.

Melatonin production can be suppressed by light, beta blockers and nonsteroidal antiinflammatory medications.[102,103,106] In addition to affecting the levels of melatonin excretion,[107] light exposure at certain times can also shift (phase advance or delay[4,5,107]) the timing of the melatonin rhythm and as such it is useful, when possible, to also assess the habitual light exposure patterns (see earlier section on rest-activity rhythms) of patients before and during the sampling period. The benefits of monitoring light levels during this time are 2-fold, one is that you can determine whether the measure is compromised and the other is that it may provide insight on how to target instructions for adjusting habitual light exposure, which is part of the clinical management of CRSWD.[10] For example, avoiding bright light at key times that may adversely affect circadian timing and seeking out light at times that may strengthen or positively affect circadian timing are a first line of clinical management for CRSWDs.[10]

Although there are several commercially available melatonin assays, the determination of melatonin levels is not a standard test performed by most clinical laboratories. Even with access to a qualified laboratory, the number of samples typically collected each day make it cost prohibitive to assay samples from a single person at a time. Currently in most clinical scenarios, there would be no more than 25 to 30 samples collected per person/day, even when 24-hour sampling is undertaken. There are companies that can provide relatively speedy turnaround (7–10 days) to assay samples for melatonin (the speed is a function of the volume of samples that they routinely process).[108]

The most commonly used marker of circadian timing taken from serial melatonin sampling is the DLMO. There are several agreed-on methods for determining DLMO using plasma and salivary melatonin levels; examples of these for plasma and salivary melatonin are provided in **Fig. 4**. For the most part the main difference for the salivary melatonin level calculation of DLMO is the absolute threshold used; while the cutoff for plasma is 10 pg/mL, the levels of melatonin detected in saliva are generally less than in plasma[109] and as such the saliva absolute threshold is typically 3 pg/mL.[110] In addition

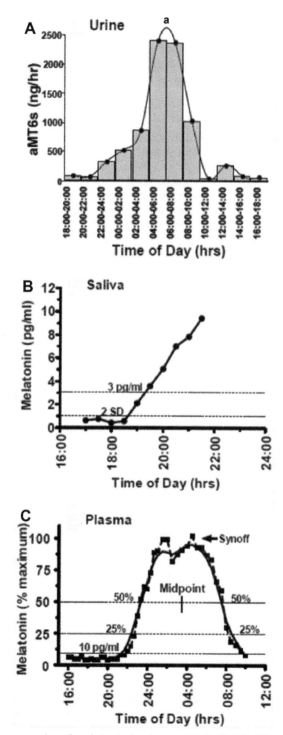

Fig. 4. Illustrative examples of melatonin levels measured using 3 different methods and their associated phase estimates. (*A*) Twenty-four–hour rhythm of primary melatonin metabolite 6-sulphatoxymelatonin (aMT6s) derived from urine samples collected in 2-hour bins

to the DLMO that only requires sampling for 5 to 6 hours, there are other markers of the melatonin rhythm that are used when sampling covers the entire melatonin profile (typically requiring sampling for 18–24 hours). The additional measures (see **Fig. 4**) include the melatonin offset (decline in circulating melatonin levels following the end of pineal production of melatonin) and midpoint of melatonin production (midpoint between the onset and offset).

Determination of the DLMO or the 24-hour rhythm of aMT6s is recommended to confirm diagnosis of various CRSWDs, including delayed sleep-wake phase disorder, advanced sleep-wake phase disorder, and non-24-hour sleep-wake rhythm disorder.[1] For both advanced and delayed sleep-wake phase disorders a single measurement of circadian phase is sufficient, but for non-24-hour sleep-wake rhythm disorder measurement at 2 time points 2 to 4 weeks apart is recommended to observe the drift in timing of the circadian clock, a key feature of this disorder.[1]

Plasma melatonin levels are typically the gold standard for assessment of circadian rhythms for research purposes but in the clinical setting it is less practical due to the need to draw serial blood samples. Usually, serial sampling requires insertion of an indwelling catheter for the duration of the sampling period. There also need to be access to a centrifuge and freezer to be able to process the samples quickly, to maintain sample integrity. All of these factors mean that it is not practical to measure melatonin from plasma at home. Although, a benefit of collecting plasma, saliva, or urine samples in the laboratory is that the environment can be controlled to minimize the impact of light on melatonin production.

Validation of at-home salivary melatonin collection for assessment of DLMO has been conducted.[108,111,112] These studies compared at-home salivary melatonin collection for calculating DLMO with DLMO determined from saliva samples collected in the laboratory.[108,111] Measuring melatonin levels at home from saliva requires the patient to carefully follow the instructions for sample collection. Instructions typically include remaining in dim light (preferably <20 lux) throughout the sampling period, not eating or drinking 10 to 15 minutes before each sample, and collecting an adequate volume of saliva. A benefit to saliva sampling is that melatonin levels in saliva are quite stable and can be stored at home until they can be returned to the laboratory for assay.

Selecting the appropriate sampling duration and frequency for the patient population you wish to assess is essential. For most people with conventional sleep-wake timing, melatonin production occurs at night and on average, the DLMO occurs 2 to 3 hours before habitual bedtime.[113] By knowing when sleep-wake occurs, you can predict the best time window for saliva sampling in most people. But in patients with circadian sleep-wake phase disorders who may not have regular sleep-wake schedules (ie, non-24-hour sleep-wake phase disorder, irregular sleep-wake phase

---

under dim light. The fitted curve reveals a significant 24-hour rhythm with maximum levels observed between 04:00 AM and 08:00 AM (ª P<.01). (B) Salivary melatonin profile collected under dim light conditions. The low threshold DLMO was defined as either the first sample to exceed and remain above a threshold of 3 pg/mL or that was 2 standard deviation (SD) above the mean of the first 3 baseline samples (2 SD). (C) Overnight plasma melatonin profile, plotted as a percentage of maximum (*dashed line*) and smoothed with a LOESS curve fit to the raw data (*solid line*). Some frequently used phase markers are shown: DLMO at 10 pg/mL, DLMO or dim light melatonin offset at 25% or 50% of maximum levels, the midpoint, and the termination of melatonin synthesis (Synoff). (*From* Benloucif S, Burgess HJ, Klerman EB, et al. Measuring melatonin in humans. J Clin Sleep Med 2008;4:66-9; with permission.)

disorder, or shift work disorder), the timing of sleep-wake and therefore melatonin onset may not be as predictable and because of this sampling needs to be tailored.[114] Examples of saliva melatonin sampling from a clinical setting are provided here to illustrate a few key concepts. In **Fig. 5**, the top panel is an example of melatonin levels from a traditional saliva sampling protocol used for the determination of DLMO. In this

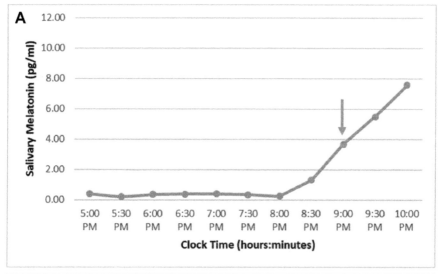

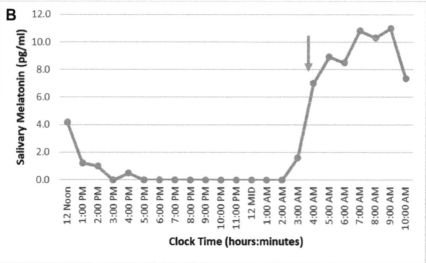

Fig. 5. Salivary melatonin levels for (A) 5 hours before bedtime and (B) 22 hours of sampling. The top panel (A) represents an example from a single individual using a common method for sampling salivary melatonin levels at home. This includes 11 total samples each taken at 30-minute intervals for the 5 hours before habitual bedtime. DLMO was calculated using the 2 SD threshold and occurred at 8:30 PM; if the 3 pg/mL threshold method is used the DLMO would be reported as 9:00 PM (indicated by the *arrow*). The bottom panel (B) represents an example for an individual who collected samples hourly for 22 hours. DLMO for this individual occurred at 3:00 AM using the 2 SD criteria or at 4:00 AM if using the 3 pg/mL threshold criteria (indicated by the *arrow*).

example, saliva samples were taken at 30-minute intervals for the 5 hours before habitual bedtime under dim light conditions and there is a clear and consistent increase in melatonin levels, such that, the DLMO onset was determined to be at 9:00 PM The lower panel of **Fig. 5** depicts a longer sampling duration (22 hours) and reduced sampling frequency (hourly) that might be used if you were not sure when the DLMO might be within the 24-hour day, such as in a patent with non-24-hour sleep-wake phase disorder. In this example, the DLMO is at around 4:00 AM

Even when you have considered all of the right factors and you have provided clear instructions to the patient you may not be able to determine the DLMO at all, an example of just such a case is provided in **Fig. 6**. In this case, it was not possible to determine whether the timing of the sample collection resulted in simply missing DLMO altogether (DLMO occurred earlier or later) or whether the individual did not follow the instructions for sample collection (ie, they did not dim lights during the collection period, which would suppress melatonin production[108,115]).

Measurement of urinary aMT6s can be useful in some instances for assessment of circadian rhythm function. It is particularly useful if you want to monitor aMT6s over many days or if you want to assess melatonin levels in infants and small children or adults with dementia. From a methodological standpoint, although urine sampling is less invasive than blood sampling, the frequency of urine sampling is less controlled, as most people cannot urinate on command. However, samples from key time periods across the day can be used to estimate a 24-hour profile of aMT6s excretion.

For 24-hour urine collection, the subject is typically instructed to void their bladder on awakening on the day of collection and discard the first void. For the next 24 hours, each void is collected in a separate container and marked with the time and date, with the final sample consisting of the first void the following morning. All samples are kept on ice after collection and brought to the laboratory the following day. In the laboratory the total volume of each void is recorded, and an aliquot of each sample is frozen for further analysis. At least 4 samples are needed for analysis of circadian parameters, which include samples from the morning, afternoon, evening, and first morning void the following day. aMT6s levels need to be adjusted with total urine volume or

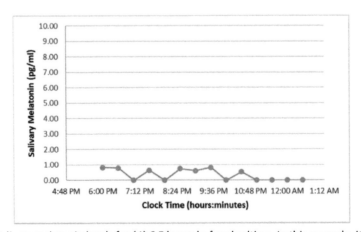

Fig. 6. Salivary melatonin levels for (A) 6.5 hours before bedtime. In this example, it was not possible to calculate the DLMO, as there was no clearly discernible melatonin levels measured. It is unclear in this case whether the DLMO was simply missed altogether or whether the individual did not follow the instructions for sample collection (ie, they did not dim lights, which would suppress melatonin production).

creatinine levels.[110,116,117] Twenty-four–hour profiles of aMT6s (see **Fig. 4**) can be analyzed using a cosinor analysis[110] to determine variables such as mesor (average of samples in the analysis), acrophase (time of peak concentration), and amplitude (difference between the acrophase and mesor).

Overnight aMT6s excretion rates or levels can also be calculated from a single morning urine sample on waking.[110,116,117] In shift workers aMT6s levels in urine from pooled samples collected during sleep and on waking from each sleep period over many days have been shown to be associated with sleep quality and sleep duration, such that when aMT6s levels are high, sleep quality and duration become better.[118]

BODY TEMPERATURE

In humans the circadian rhythm of CBT has been used to assess the timing of the circadian system and for many years was the most commonly used method. Typically the nadir of the CBT rhythm is used as a marker of circadian phase. With the discovery of melatonin and development of melatonin collection and assay methods, a shift has occurred toward melatonin as the circadian marker of choice. The reason for this shift, at least in part, stems from the masking effects of activity and meals on core body temperate and that measurement of CBT was usually collected via a probe inserted into the rectum.[119,120] Even with these caveats, the circadian rhythm of CBT is a useful measure of circadian rhythms and is particularly useful if you want to determine circadian timing quickly and not have to wait for the return of assay results, which typically require a minimum 7- to 10-day turnaround. Furthermore, there have been technological advances that provide options for measuring CBT such as devices that can be swallowed and transmit real time temperature data as they pass through the digestive tract.[121]

CBT is closely linked with sleep-wake,[31] and CBT nadir typically occurs during the latter part of the habitual sleep period in those with conventional sleep times (ie, around 3–4 AM). However, in those with a CRSWD the CBT can be at an earlier or later clock time[60] or even outside of the normal sleep-wake period as would be commonly seen in shift workers.[122] The profile of the CBT rhythm is typically the opposite of the melatonin rhythm. Although melatonin levels are high during the biological night, CBT is low. The ability to fall asleep is typically greatest when core temperature levels are declining. In addition, administration of exogenous melatonin during the day when melatonin levels are typically low and CBT is high can also acutely reduce CBT levels and increase sleepiness.[120]

An example of a 24-hour profile of CBT from a patient with delayed sleep-wake phase disorder is shown in **Fig. 7**; in this case the CBT nadir was at 9 AM The 24-hour CBT profile shown here was quantitatively described using the Cleveland regression procedure to assess the phase of the rhythm.[123]

Skin temperature can also be used as a marker of circadian timing.[124,125] Although this method is much less invasive than measures of CBT, interpretation of temperature profiles using this method should be used with caution, as ambient temperature, location of the sensors, and activity level can substantially influence the measurement. Something to note about skin temperature is that it is typically higher during the sleep period (**Fig. 8**), compared with CBT, which is lower during sleep (see **Fig. 7**). There are several commercially available devices that measure skin temperature including small battery–sized devices[121] that can be taped to the skin or a wrist-worn device available that integrates skin temperature, activity, and light level measurement.[126] An example of data from such an integrated device is provided in **Fig. 8**.

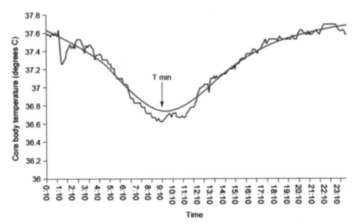

Fig. 7. Twenty-four–hour recording of CBT. This is an example of a 24-hour recording of rectal temperature from a patient with delayed sleep-wake phase disorder. Clock time (hours:minutes) is indicated on the x-axis and temperature (degrees Celsius) on the y-axis. The raw temperature data are indicated by the blue line, whereas the pink line indicates the fitted curve for the calculation of CBT minimum. The calculated CBT is indicated by the *black arrow* and was at 9 AM. The declining portion of the CBT rhythm begins at about 3 AM and the rising potion of the rhythm occurs at 11 AM. This would make it difficult for this person to fall asleep earlier than 3 AM and wake before 11 AM and if they did wake at 11 AM they would likely report feeling very sleepy as the CBT is still low. (*From* Reid KJ, Zee PC. Circadian Rhythm Sleep Disorders. In: Kryger M, ed. Atlas of Clinical Sleep Medicine. 2nd ed: Saunder, Elsevier, 2013; with permission.)

THE FUTURE

Assessment of circadian rhythms in humans has been and continues to be challenging. As our knowledge about the complexities of the circadian system and the technologies to measure these systems advance, there have been exciting developments in potential new markers of the circadian system that may soon be transferable to the clinical environment.

With the discovery that almost all cells of the body contain the genetic components of the clock and development of new technologies, the methods to assess circadian rhythms have expanded. For example, we are no longer limited to measuring circadian

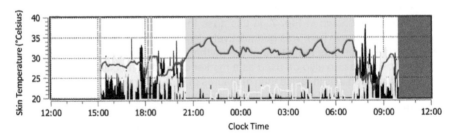

Fig. 8. An example of activity, light, and skin temperature levels with a wrist-worn device between 3 PM–10 AM Activity levels are indicated in blue, light levels in yellow and skin temperature in red. The light blue shaded area indicates the sleep period. In contrast to CBT, skin temperature is higher during the sleep period when core temperature is normally lower.

rhythm outputs in humans but we can also measure the rhythms of the bacteria that live within them. It is thought that these bacteria may influence the function of the brain, gut, and other systems within the body.[127] We can also measure circadian expression of core clock and other genes in peripheral blood mononuclear cells; a limitation of this technology has been that it still requires serial sampling for 24-hours or more. However, there are several groups working on techniques and analytical methods to limit the number of blood samples that are required to accurately determine circadian rhythms.[128–133]

We also have a better understanding of how external stimuli (zeitgebers) influence the circadian system, and how the systems that relay this information to the SCN can be altered in various patient populations. As an example pupilometry is being used to determine the responsiveness of the retina to light stimuli; although this is not a direct measure of circadian rhythms, it has implications for how the external environment interfaces with the circadian clock to affect circadian rhythms. A recent publication in those with DSWPD suggests that there is potential for the pupillary light reflex to clinically differentiate between DSWPD patients with normal versus delayed circadian timing relative to desired bedtime, without the need for costly and time-consuming circadian assessments.[8]

Finally, it is also becoming clearer that circadian disturbance is not limited to those who meet the criteria for CRSWDs.[59] Because of our 24/7 lifestyle and the shifting of the sleep-wake period from day-to-day and from weekday-weekends, even this seemly benign level of circadian disruption if extreme enough can result in poor mental and physical health outcomes.[11,39,41–45,59,68,134,135] In fact, circadian disturbance itself may be a risk factor or a marker for disease severity or even a marker for eventual progression to disease.

SUMMARY

As the role the circadian system plays in health and safety is better understood, the need to assess circadian rhythms has expanded. Even current methods of assessing circadian rhythms are not readily available to the average physician for use in the management of patients with circadian rhythm disturbance; rather, they are relegated to the research environment. Translation of currently available methods of assessing circadian rhythms to the clinical environment and development of new simple and cost-effective methods for the assessment of circadian rhythms will be essential for the future of circadian medicine.

ACKNOWLEDGMENTS

Dr Reid was supported by National Institutes of Health grants R01 HL140580-01 and P01 AG011412-18A1.

A special thank you to Dr Sabra M. Abbott MD, PhD for salivary melatonin profiles from her clinical population and to Dr Daniela Grimaldi MD, PhD for reviewing a copy of this article.

REFERENCES

1. Sateia M. International classification of sleep disorders. 3rd edition. Darien (IL): American Acadmey of Sleep Medicine; 2014.

2. Vitaterna MH, Takahashi JS, Turek FW. Overview of circadian rhythms. Alcohol Res Health 2001;25:85–93.

3. Burgess HJ, Revell VL, Molina TA, et al. Human phase response curves to three days of daily melatonin: 0.5 mg versus 3.0 mg. J Clin Endocrinol Metab 2010;95: 3325–31.

4. Khalsa SB, Jewett ME, Cajochen C, et al. A phase response curve to single bright light pulses in human subjects. J Physiol 2003;549:945–52.

5. Kim SJ, Benloucif S, Reid KJ, et al. Phase-shifting response to light in older adults. J Physiol 2014;592:189–202.

6. Ruger M, St Hilaire MA, Brainard GC, et al. Human phase response curve to a single 6.5 h pulse of short-wavelength light. J Physiol 2013;591:353–63.

7. St Hilaire MA, Gooley JJ, Khalsa SB, et al. Human phase response curve to a 1 h pulse of bright white light. J Physiol 2012;590:3035–45.

8. McGlashan EM, Burns AC, Murray JM, et al. The pupillary light reflex distinguishes between circadian and non-circadian delayed sleep phase disorder (DSPD) phenotypes in young adults. PLoS One 2018;13:e0204621.

9. Murray JM, Sletten TL, Magee M, et al. Prevalence of circadian misalignment and its association with depressive symptoms in delayed sleep phase disorder. Sleep 2017;40. https://doi.org/10.1093/sleep/zsw002.

10. Auger RR, Burgess HJ, Emens JS, et al. Clinical practice guideline for the treatment of intrinsic circadian rhythm sleep-wake disorders: advanced sleep-wake phase disorder (ASWPD), delayed sleep-wake phase disorder (DSWPD), Non-24-Hour sleep-wake rhythm disorder (N24SWD), and irregular sleep-wake rhythm disorder (ISWRD). an update for 2015: an American Academy of Sleep Medicine clinical practice guideline. J Clin Sleep Med 2015;11:1199–236.

11. Abbott SM, Malkani RG, Zee PC. Circadian disruption and human health: a bidirectional relationship. Eur J Neurosci 2018. https://doi.org/10.1111/ejn.14298.

12. Edgar D. Circadian control of sleep/wakefulness: implications in shiftwork and therapeutic strategies. In: Shiraki K, Sagawa S, Yousef MK, editors. Physiological basis of occupational health: stressful environments. Amsterdam: Academic Publishing; 1996. p. 253–65.

13. Edgar D. Functional role of the suprachiasmatic nuclei in the regulation of sleep and wakefulness. In: Guilleminault C, Lugaresi E, Montagna P, et al, editors. Fatal familial insomnia: inherited prion diseases, sleep, and the thalamus. New York: Raven Press; 1994. p. 203–13.

14. Meijer JH, Rietveld WJ. Neurophysiology of the suprachiasmatic circadian pacemaker in rodents. Physiol Rev 1989;69:671–707.

15. Mistlberger R, Rusak B. Mechanisms and models of the circadian timekeeping system. In: Kryger M, Roth T, Dement W, editors. Principles and practice of sleep medicine. Philadelphia: W.B. Saunders Company; 1989. p. 141–52.

16. Moore-Ede MCS, Sulzman F, Fuller C. The clocks that time us. Cambridge: Harvard University Press; 1982.

17. Klein DC, Moore RY. Pineal N-acetyltransferase and hydroxyindole-O-methyltransferase: control by the retinohypothalamic tract and the suprachiasmatic nucleus. Brain Res 1979;174:245–62.

18. Harrington ME. The ventral lateral geniculate nucleus and the intergeniculate leaflet: interrelated structures in the visual and circadian systems. Neurosci Biobehav Rev 1997;21:705–27.

19. Freedman MS, Lucas RJ, Soni B, et al. Regulation of mammalian circadian behavior by non-rod, non-cone, ocular photoreceptors. Science 1999;284: 502–4.

20. Ruby NF, Brennan TJ, Xie X, et al. Role of melanopsin in circadian responses to light. Science 2002;298:2211–3.

21. Lockley SW, Brainard GC, Czeisler CA. High sensitivity of the human circadian melatonin rhythm to resetting by short wavelength light. J Clin Endocrinol Metab 2003;88:4502–5.
22. Warman VL, Dijk DJ, Warman GR, et al. Phase advancing human circadian rhythms with short wavelength light. Neurosci Lett 2003;342:37–40.
23. Buxton OM, Frank SA, L'Hermite-Baleriaux M, et al. Roles of intensity and duration of nocturnal exercise in causing phase delays of human circadian rhythms. Am J Physiol 1997;273:E536–42.
24. Van Reeth O, Sturis J, Byrne MM, et al. Nocturnal exercise phase delays circadian rhythms of melatonin and thyrotropin secretion in normal men. Am J Physiol 1994;266:E964–74.
25. Borbely AA. Sleep: circadian rhythm vs. recovery process. In: Koukkou ML, D. Angst J, editors. Functional states of the brain: the determinants. Amsterdam: Elsevier/North-Holland; 1980. p. 151–62.
26. Borbely AA. A two process model of sleep regulation. Hum Neurobiol 1982;1: 195–204.
27. Czeisler CA, Weitzman E, Moore-Ede MC, et al. Human sleep: its duration and organization depend on its circadian phase. Science 1980;210:1264–7.
28. Dijk DJ, Czeisler CA. Paradoxical timing of the circadian rhythm of sleep propensity serves to consolidate sleep and wakefulness in humans. Neurosci Lett 1994;166:63–8.
29. Edgar DM, Dement WC, Fuller CA. Effect of SCN lesions on sleep in squirrel monkeys: evidence for opponent processes in sleep-wake regulation. J Neurosci 1993;13:1065–79.
30. Wever R. The circadian system of man. New York: Springer-Verlag; 1979.
31. Zulley J, Wever R, Aschoff J. The dependence of onset and duration of sleep on the circadian rhythm of rectal temperature. Pflugers Arch 1981;391:314–8.
32. Carskadon MA, Dement WC. Sleepiness and sleep state on a 90-min schedule. Psychophysiology 1977;14:127–33.
33. Carskadon MA, Dement W. Sleep studies on a 90-minute day. Electroencephalogr Clin Neurophysiol 1975;39:145–55.
34. Dantz B, Edgar DM, Dement WC. Circadian rhythms in narcolepsy: studies on a 90 minute day. Electroencephalogr Clin Neurophysiol 1994;90:24–35.
35. Dijk DJ, Czeisler CA. Contribution of the circadian pacemaker and the sleep homeostat to sleep propensity, sleep structure, electroencephalographic slow waves, and sleep spindle activity in humans. J Neurosci 1995;15:3526–38.
36. Strogatz SH, Kronauer RE, Czeisler CA. Circadian pacemaker interferes with sleep onset at specific times each day: role in insomnia. Am J Physiol 1987; 253:R172–8.
37. Dijk DJ, Beersma DG, van den Hoofdakker RH. All night spectral analysis of EEG sleep in young adult and middle-aged male subjects. Neurobiol Aging 1989;10:677–82.
38. Dijk DJ, Brunner DP, Beersma DG, et al. Electroencephalogram power density and slow wave sleep as a function of prior waking and circadian phase. Sleep 1990;13:430–40.
39. Abbott SM, Weng J, Reid KJ, et al. Sleep timing, stability, and BP in the sueno ancillary study of the hispanic community health study/study of latinos. Chest 2019;155:60–8.
40. Baron KG, Reid KJ. Relationship between circdian rhyhtms, feeding and obesity. In: Watson R, editor. Modulation of sleep by obesity, diabetes, age and diet. London: Elsevier; 2015. p. 141–52.

41. Facco FL, Grobman WA, Reid KJ, et al. Objectively measured short sleep duration and later sleep midpoint in pregnancy are associated with a higher risk of gestational diabetes. Am J Obstet Gynecol 2017;217(4):447.e1-e13.

42. Baron KG, Reid KJ, Kim T, et al. Circadian timing and alignment in healthy adults: associations with BMI, body fat, caloric intake and physical activity. Int J Obes (Lond) 2017;41:203–9.

43. Baron KG, Reid KJ, Wolfe LF, et al. Phase relationship between DLMO and sleep onset and the risk of metabolic disease among normal weight and overweight/obese adults. J Biol Rhythms 2018;33:76–83.

44. McHill AW, Czeisler CA, Phillips AJK, et al. Caloric and macronutrient intake differ with circadian phase and between lean and overweight young adults. Nutrients 2019;11 [pii:E587].

45. McHill AW, Phillips AJ, Czeisler CA, et al. Later circadian timing of food intake is associated with increased body fat. Am J Clin Nutr 2017;106:1213–9.

46. Czeisler CA, Duffy JF, Shanahan TL, et al. Stability, precision, and near-24-hour period of the human circadian pacemaker. Science 1999;284:2177–81.

47. Dijk DJ, Duffy JF, Riel E, et al. Ageing and the circadian and homeostatic regulation of human sleep during forced desynchrony of rest, melatonin and temperature rhythms. J Physiol 1999;516(Pt 2):611–27.

48. Duffy JF, Dijk DJ. Getting through to circadian oscillators: why use constant routines? J Biol Rhythms 2002;17:4–13.

49. Medicine AAoS. Two week sleep diary. Available at: http://yoursleep.aasmnet.org/pdf/sleepdiary.pdf. Accessed April 29, 2019.

50. Horne JA, Ostberg O. A self-assessment questionnaire to determine morningness-eveningness in human circadian rhythms. Int J Chronobiol 1976; 4:97–110.

51. Roenneberg T, Wirz-Justice A, Merrow M. Life between clocks: daily temporal patterns of human chronotypes. J Biol Rhythms 2003;18:80–90.

52. Zavada A, Gordijn MC, Beersma DG, et al. Comparison of the Munich chronotype questionnaire with the Horne-Ostberg's Morningness-Eveningness score. Chronobiol Int 2005;22:267–78.

53. Juda M, Vetter C, Roenneberg T. The Munich chronotype questionnaire for shift-workers (MCTQShift). J Biol Rhythms 2013;28:130–40.

54. Andrade MM, Benedito-Silva AA, Menna-Barreto L. Correlations between morningness-eveningness character, sleep habits and temperature rhythm in adolescents. Braz J Med Biol Res 1992;25:835–9.

55. Baehr EK, Revelle W, Eastman CI. Individual differences in the phase and amplitude of the human circadian temperature rhythm: with an emphasis on morningness-eveningness. J Sleep Res 2000;9:117–27.

56. Breithaupt H, Hildebrandt G, Werner A. Circadian type questionnaire and objective circadian characteristics. In: Reinberg A, Vieux N, Andlauer P, editors. Night and shift work: biological and social aspects. Oxford (England): Pergamon Press; 1981. p. 435–40.

57. Folkard S, Monk T. Shiftwork and performance. Hum Factors 1979;21:483–92.

58. Waterhouse J, Folkard S, Van Dongen H, et al. Temperature profiles, and the effect of sleep on them, in relation to morningness-eveningness in healthy female subjects. Chronobiol Int 2001;18:227–47.

59. Wittmann M, Dinich J, Merrow M, et al. Social jetlag: misalignment of biological and social time. Chronobiol Int 2006;23:497–509.

60. Chang AM, Reid KJ, Gourineni R, et al. Sleep timing and circadian phase in delayed sleep phase syndrome. J Biol Rhythms 2009;24:313–21.

61. Wilson Jt, Reid KJ, Braun RI, et al. Habitual light exposure relative to circadian timing in delayed sleep-wake phase disorder. Sleep 2018;41. https://doi.org/10.1093/sleep/zsy166.
62. Reid KJ, Chang AM, Dubocovich ML, et al. Familial advanced sleep phase syndrome. Arch Neurol 2001;58:1089–94.
63. Foret J, Benoit O, Royant-Parola S. Sleep schedules and peak times of oral temperature and alertness in morning and evening 'types'. Ergonomics 1982;25:821–7.
64. Webb WB, Bonnet MH. The sleep of 'morning' and 'evening' types. Biol Psychol 1978;7:29–35.
65. Breithaupt H, Hildebrandt G, Dohre D, et al. Tolerance to shift of sleep, as related to the individual's circadian phase position. Ergonomics 1978;21:767–74.
66. Mongrain V, Carrier J, Dumont M. Difference in sleep regulation between morning and evening circadian types as indexed by antero-posterior analyses of the sleep EEG. Eur J Neurosci 2006;23:497–504.
67. Mongrain V, Lavoie S, Selmaoui B, et al. Phase relationships between sleep-wake cycle and underlying circadian rhythms in Morningness-Eveningness. J Biol Rhythms 2004;19:248–57.
68. Roenneberg T, Allebrandt KV, Merrow M, et al. Social jetlag and obesity. Curr Biol 2012;22:939–43.
69. Roenneberg T, Kuehnle T, Juda M, et al. Epidemiology of the human circadian clock. Sleep Med Rev 2007;11:429–38.
70. Ancoli-Israel S, Cole R, Alessi C, et al. The role of actigraphy in the study of sleep and circadian rhythms. Sleep 2003;26:342–92.
71. Ancoli-Israel S, Martin JL, Blackwell T, et al. The SBSM guide to actigraphy monitoring: clinical and research applications. Behav Sleep Med 2015;13(Suppl 1):S4–38.
72. Smith MT, McCrae CS, Cheung J, et al. Use of actigraphy for the evaluation of sleep disorders and circadian rhythm sleep-wake disorders: an american academy of sleep medicine systematic review, meta-analysis, and GRADE assessment. J Clin Sleep Med 2018;14:1209–30.
73. Smith MT, McCrae CS, Cheung J, et al. Use of actigraphy for the evaluation of sleep disorders and circadian rhythm sleep-wake disorders: an American Academy of Sleep Medicine clinical practice guideline. J Clin Sleep Med 2018;14:1231–7.
74. Sack RL, Lewy AJ, Blood ML, et al. Circadian rhythm abnormalities in totally blind people: incidence and clinical significance. J Clin Endocrinol Metab 1992;75:127–34.
75. Maglione JE, Ancoli-Israel S, Peters KW, et al. Depressive symptoms and circadian activity rhythm disturbances in community-dwelling older women. Am J Geriatr Psychiatry 2014;22:349–61.
76. Paudel ML, Taylor BC, Ancoli-Israel S, et al. Rest/activity rhythms and mortality rates in older men: MrOS Sleep Study. Chronobiol Int 2010;27:363–77.
77. Paudel ML, Taylor BC, Ancoli-Israel S, et al. Rest/activity rhythms and cardiovascular disease in older men. Chronobiol Int 2011;28:258–66.
78. Tranah GJ, Blackwell T, Ancoli-Israel S, et al. Circadian activity rhythms and mortality: the study of osteoporotic fractures. J Am Geriatr Soc 2010;58:282–91.
79. Reid KJ, Facco FL, Grobman WA, et al. Sleep during pregnancy: the nuMoM2b pregnancy and sleep duration and Continuity Study. Sleep 2017;40. https://doi.org/10.1093/sleep/zsx045.

80. Boubekri M, Cheung IN, Reid KJ, et al. Impact of windows and daylight exposure on overall health and sleep quality of office workers: a case-control pilot study. J Clin Sleep Med 2014;10:603–11.

81. Cheung IN, Zee PC, Shalman D, et al. Morning and evening blue-enriched light exposure alters metabolic function in normal weight adults. PLoS One 2016;11: e0155601.

82. Reid KJ, Santostasi G, Baron KG, et al. Timing and intensity of light correlate with body weight in adults. PLoS One 2014;9:e92251.

83. Auger RR, Burgess HJ, Dierkhising RA, et al. Light exposure among adolescents with delayed sleep phase disorder: a prospective cohort study. Chronobiol Int 2011;28:911–20.

84. Joo EY, Abbott SM, Reid KJ, et al. Timing of light exposure and activity in adults with delayed sleep-wake phase disorder. Sleep Med 2017;32:259–65.

85. Marler MR, Gehrman P, Martin JL, et al. The sigmoidally transformed cosine curve: a mathematical model for circadian rhythms with symmetric non-sinusoidal shapes. Stat Med 2006;25:3893–904.

86. Tranah GJ, Blackwell T, Stone KL, et al. Circadian activity rhythms and risk of incident dementia and mild cognitive impairment in older women. Ann Neurol 2011;70:722–32.

87. Rogers TS, Blackwell TL, Lane NE, et al. Rest-activity patterns and falls and fractures in older men. Osteoporos Int 2017;28:1313–22.

88. Rogers-Soeder TS, Blackwell T, Yaffe K, et al. Rest-activity rhythms and cognitive decline in older men: the osteoporotic fractures in men sleep study. J Am Geriatr Soc 2018;66:2136–43.

89. Ancoli-Israel S, Liu L, Marler MR, et al. Fatigue, sleep, and circadian rhythms prior to chemotherapy for breast cancer. Support Care Cancer 2006;14:201–9.

90. van Someren EJ, Hagebeuk EE, Lijzenga C, et al. Circadian rest-activity rhythm disturbances in Alzheimer's disease. Biol Psychiatry 1996;40:259–70.

91. Witting W, Kwa IH, Eikelenboom P, et al. Alterations in the circadian rest-activity rhythm in aging and Alzheimer's disease. Biol Psychiatry 1990;27:563–72.

92. Blume C, Santhi N, Schabus M. 'nparACT' package for R: a free software tool for the non-parametric analysis of actigraphy data. MethodsX 2016;3:430–5.

93. Cavalcanti-Ferreira P, Berk L, Daher N, et al. A nonparametric methodological analysis of rest-activity rhythm in type 2 diabetes. Sleep Sci 2018;11:281–9.

94. Lerner AB, Case JD, Takahashi Y, et al. Isolation of melatonin, the pineal gland factor that lightens melanocytes. J Am Chem Soc 1958;80:2587.

95. Moore RY. Neural control of the pineal gland. Behav Brain Res 1996;73:125–30.

96. Moore RY. Suprachiasmatic nucleus in sleep-wake regulation. Sleep Med 2007; 8(Suppl 3):27–33.

97. Burgess HJ, Revell VL, Eastman CI. A three pulse phase response curve to three milligrams of melatonin in humans. J Physiol 2008;586:639–47.

98. Lewy AL, Ahmed S, Jackson JML, et al. Melatonin shifts human circadian rhythms according to a phase-response curve. Chronobiol Int 1992;9:380–92.

99. Jin X, von Gall C, Pieschl RL, et al. Targeted disruption of the mouse Mel(1b) melatonin receptor. Mol Cell Biol 2003;23:1054–60.

100. Liu C, Weaver DR, Jin X, et al. Molecular dissection of two distinct actions of melatonin on the suprachiasmatic circadian clock. Neuron 1997;19:91–102.

101. Murphy DL, Garrick NA, Tamarkin L, et al. Effects of antidepressants and other psychotropic drugs on melatonin release and pineal gland function. J Neural Transm Suppl 1986;21:291–309.

102. Murphy PJ, Myers BL, Badia P. Nonsteroidal anti-inflammatory drugs alter body temperature and suppress melatonin in humans. Physiol Behav 1996;59:133–9.

103. Van Den Heuvel CJ, Reid KJ, Dawson D. Effect of atenolol on nocturnal sleep and temperature in young men: reversal by pharmacological doses of melatonin. Physiol Behav 1997;61:795–802.

104. Montagnese S, Middleton B, Mani AR, et al. Melatonin rhythms in patients with cirrhosis. Am J Gastroenterol 2010;105:220–2 [author reply 2].

105. Videnovic A, Noble C, Reid KJ, et al. Circadian melatonin rhythm and excessive daytime sleepiness in Parkinson disease. JAMA Neurol 2014;71:463–9.

106. Czeisler CA, Shanahan TL, Klerman EB, et al. Suppression of melatonin secretion in some blind patients by exposure to bright light. N Engl J Med 1995; 332:6–11.

107. Lewy AJ. Effects of light on human melatonin production and the human circadian system. Prog Neuropsychopharmacol Biol Psychiatry 1983;7:551–6.

108. Burgess HJ, Wyatt JK, Park M, et al. Home circadian phase assessments with measures of compliance yield accurate dim light melatonin onsets. Sleep 2015;38:889–97.

109. Voultsios A, Kennaway DJ, Dawson D. Salivary melatonin as a circadian phase marker: validation and comparison to plasma melatonin. J Biol Rhythms 1997; 12:457–66.

110. Benloucif S, Burgess HJ, Klerman EB, et al. Measuring melatonin in humans. J Clin Sleep Med 2008;4:66–9.

111. Burgess HJ, Park M, Wyatt JK, et al. Home dim light melatonin onsets with measures of compliance in delayed sleep phase disorder. J Sleep Res 2016;25: 314–7.

112. Pullman RE, Roepke SE, Duffy JF. Laboratory validation of an in-home method for assessing circadian phase using dim light melatonin onset (DLMO). Sleep Med 2012;13:703–6.

113. Burgess HJ, Savic N, Sletten T, et al. The relationship between the dim light melatonin onset and sleep on a regular schedule in young healthy adults. Behav Sleep Med 2003;1:102–14.

114. Malkani RG, Abbott SM, Reid KJ, et al. Diagnostic and treatment challenges of sighted non-24-hour sleep-wake disorder. J Clin Sleep Med 2018;14:603–13.

115. Lewy AJ, Wehr TA, Goodwin FK, et al. Light suppresses melatonin secretion in humans. Science 1980;210:1267–9.

116. Cook MR, Graham C, Kavet R, et al. Morning urinary assessment of nocturnal melatonin secretion in older women. J Pineal Res 2000;28:41–7.

117. Graham C, Cook MR, Kavet R, et al. Prediction of nocturnal plasma melatonin from morning urinary measures. J Pineal Res 1998;24:230–8.

118. Roach GD, Reid KJ, Ferguson S, et al. The relationship between the rate of melatonin excretion and sleep consolidation for locomotive engineers in natural sleep settings. J Circadian Rhythms 2006;4:8.

119. Benloucif S, Guico MJ, Reid KJ, et al. Stability of melatonin and temperature as circadian phase markers and their relation to sleep times in humans. J Biol Rhythms 2005;20:178–88.

120. Reid K, Van den Heuvel C, Dawson D. Day-time melatonin administration: effects on core temperature and sleep onset latency. J Sleep Res 1996;5:150–4.

121. Krauchi K, Fattori E, Giordano A, et al. Sleep on a high heat capacity mattress increases conductive body heat loss and slow wave sleep. Physiol Behav 2018; 185:23–30.

122. Smith MR, Eastman CI. Night shift performance is improved by a compromise circadian phase position: study 3. Circadian phase after 7 night shifts with an intervening weekend off. Sleep 2008;31:1639–45.

123. Cleveland WS. Robust locally weighted regression and smoothing scatterplots. J Am Stat Assoc 1979;74:829–36.

124. Hasselberg MJ, McMahon J, Parker K. The validity, reliability, and utility of the iButton(R) for measurement of body temperature circadian rhythms in sleep/wake research. Sleep Med 2013;14:5–11.

125. Scully CG, Karaboue A, Liu WM, et al. Skin surface temperature rhythms as potential circadian biomarkers for personalized chronotherapeutics in cancer patients. Interface Focus 2011;1:48–60.

126. Bellone GJ, Plano SA, Cardinali DP, et al. Comparative analysis of actigraphy performance in healthy young subjects. Sleep Sci 2016;9:272–9.

127. Li Y, Hao Y, Fan F, et al. The role of microbiome in insomnia, circadian disturbance and depression. Front Psychiatry 2018;9:669.

128. Agostinelli F, Ceglia N, Shahbaba B, et al. What time is it? Deep learning approaches for circadian rhythms. Bioinformatics 2016;32:i8–17.

129. Braun R, Kath WL, Iwanaszko M, et al. Universal method for robust detection of circadian state from gene expression. Proc Natl Acad Sci U S A 2018;115:E9247–56.

130. Braun R, Kath WL, Iwanaszko M, et al. Reply to Laing et al.: accurate prediction of circadian time across platforms. Proc Natl Acad Sci U S A 2019;116:5206–8.

131. Hughey JJ. Machine learning identifies a compact gene set for monitoring the circadian clock in human blood. Genome Med 2017;9:19.

132. Hughey JJ, Hastie T, Butte AJ. ZeitZeiger: supervised learning for high-dimensional data from an oscillatory system. Nucleic Acids Res 2016;44:e80.

133. Laing EE, Moller-Levet CS, Poh N, et al. Blood transcriptome based biomarkers for human circadian phase. Elife 2017;6 [pii:e20214].

134. Fan EP, Abbott SM, Reid KJ, et al. Abnormal environmental light exposure in the intensive care environment. J Crit Care 2017;40:11–4.

135. Hori H, Koga N, Hidese S, et al. 24-h activity rhythm and sleep in depressed outpatients. J Psychiatr Res 2016;77:27–34.

Circadian Rhythm Sleep-Wake Phase Disorders

Elizabeth Culnan, PhD[a], Lindsay M. McCullough, MD[b], James K. Wyatt, PhD[a],*

KEYWORDS

- Circadian • Sleep homeostasis • Melatonin • Phototherapy • Chronotherapy
- Sleep disorder

KEY POINTS

- Diagnosing either delayed or advanced sleep-wake phase disorder requires a clinical interview and at least a week of sleep diary information. Objective estimation of sleep-wake patterns and/or measurement of circadian phase from the dim light melatonin onset can also aid in making the diagnosis.
- Timed, ocular exposure to bright light (phototherapy) is an evidence-based treatment for delayed sleep-wake phase disorder (DSWPD) and advanced sleep-wake phase disorder (ASWPD).
- Melatonin administration can advance circadian phase and sleep timing in patients with DSWPD, although relapse may be high after discontinuation.
- Evidence is mounting that DSWPD may share clinical features with the insomnia disorders, suggesting they may not always be entirely separate sleep disorders.

INTRODUCTION AND OVERVIEW

Delayed and advanced sleep-wake phase disorders (DSWPD and ASWPD) appeared in the literature approximately 40 years ago as delayed sleep phase syndrome[1] and advanced sleep phase syndrome.[2] They have traditionally been viewed as a misalignment of the endogenous circadian timekeeping system with the desired sleep-wake schedule. However, with consideration of the 2-process model of sleep-wake regulation,[3] these disorders clearly involve the sleep homeostatic system as well.[4] For example, those with DSWPD encounter insufficient sleep duration if enforced to a more "traditional" sleep schedule, hence homeostatic sleep pressure builds

Disclosure: Dr E. Culnan and Dr L. McCullough have no conflicts of interest to disclose. Dr J.K. Wyatt receives royalties from UpToDate.
[a] Department of Psychiatry and Behavioral Sciences, Rush University Medical Center, 1653 West Congress Parkway, Chicago, IL 60612-3833, USA; [b] Department of Medicine, Rush University Medical Center, 1653 West Congress Parkway, Chicago, IL 60612-3833, USA
* Corresponding author.
E-mail address: jwyatt@rush.edu
; @Chisleeper (J.K.W.)

incrementally and relentlessly across the work or school week. At more recent international conferences and in some publications,[5,6] there is evolving consideration that these circadian rhythm sleep-wake disorders may not be entirely distinct from the traditional insomnia disorders. What follows is foundational as well as state-of-the-art information on the diagnostic and treatment considerations for these circadian rhythm sleep-wake disorders, with subsequent future challenges in sleep and circadian medicine.

DIAGNOSTIC CRITERIA

Diagnostic criteria for circadian rhythm disorders are provided in both the International Classification for Sleep Disorders (ICSD) and the Diagnostic and Statistical Manual of Mental Disorders (DSM). Both the ICSD-3[7] and the DSM-5[8] have 3 major criteria that must be met for any Circadian Rhythm Sleep Disorder. These major criteria include (1) sleep disruption that can be attributed to disruption of the circadian system or a misalignment between an individual's endogenous rhythm and the sleep-wake schedule needed for work and social activities, which is (2) associated with daytime sleepiness and/or insomnia and (3) causes clinically significant impairment or distress in at least 1 domain of functioning (eg, social, occupational).

The DSM-5 allows for the diagnosis to be further described with a subtype of delayed sleep phase type when the sleep-wake schedule is significantly delayed or advanced sleep phase type when the sleep-wake schedule is significantly advanced.[8] Similarly, the ICSD-3 allows for a diagnosis of DSWPD when there is a significant delay in sleep-wake patterns and ASWPD when there is a significant advance in sleep-wake patterns compared with what is desired or required as reported by patient or caregiver. In contrast to the DSM-5, the ICSD-3 provides further requirements for the diagnosis, specifying that the delayed or advanced sleep-wake schedule must be present for at least 3 months, and if an individual is allowed to function on his or her preferred sleep-wake schedule, sleep quality and duration will improve but sleep-wake patterns will still be shifted. The sleep disturbance must also not be better explained by another sleep disorder, medical disorder, or psychiatric disorder.

ASSESSMENT
Traditional Assessment Strategy

Diagnosis of DSWPD and ASWPD is composed of a thorough assessment including a clinical interview and at least 1 week (7 days) of prospective, daily sleep diaries that capture both school and/or work nights, as well as free nights.[7,9] Sleep diaries, such as the Consensus Sleep Diary, have been created to standardize assessment and ensure all appropriate data about perception of sleep are captured.[10] In addition, they allow for the collection of subjective data regarding daytime functioning (eg, fatigue and sleepiness levels) and factors that may impact sleep (eg, medication use, alcohol, and caffeine intake).

Wrist actigraphy also may be recommended to complement the sleep diary data and to gather objective data of rest and activity patterns to confirm the diagnosis.[7] Actigraphy data have been found to correlate with markers of an individual's circadian phase in both ASWPD and DSWPD.[9,11] Activity data combined with the timing of morning light exposure showed very high correlation with circadian phase in patients with DSWPD.[12] The use of actigraphy is particularly useful when assessing patients who may have difficulty completing a sleep diary or who's self-report appears to be unreliable. For instance, an adolescent with suspected DSWPD who forgets to complete the sleep diary may benefit from actigraphy. Similarly, assessment of altered sleep-wake timing may be more reliably captured through actigraphy in an individual with cognitive impairment, such as an older adult with mild cognitive impairment and suspected ASWPD. **Fig. 1** displays wrist actigraphy data from a patient diagnosed with DSWPD. Visual inspection of the rest-activity patterns suggests this patient typically falls asleep for the major sleep episode in the 3 to 6 AM time period, often arising for the day after noontime. Episodic napping is also noted, as are time of bright light exposure leading close to bedtime, both factors likely worsening the delayed timing of sleep.

The clinical sleep interview, which relies on the report of the patient and/or a bed-partner or caregiver, should include information regarding the patient's sleep-wake schedule, including work days and free days.[6] Information regarding what the patient's preferred schedule would be if he or she were free to select his or her own, and how the sleep-wake patterns change when given the opportunity to function on such a schedule is also crucial for diagnosis and for differential diagnosis. For instance, individuals with DSWPD often present with complaints of sleep-onset insomnia; however, when they are able to delay bedtime and wake time to match their preferred sleep schedule, sleep-onset latency will no longer be increased. Last, clinical interview should include questions to screen for other sleep disorders, psychiatric disorders, and medical disorders that may lead to a presentation that is similar to a circadian rhythm disorder or that may exacerbate a circadian rhythm disorder. For instance, individuals with ASWPD may initially appear as if they have a disorder of excessive daytime sleepiness, given complaints of difficulties maintaining wakefulness, or depression, given complaints of early-morning awakenings.

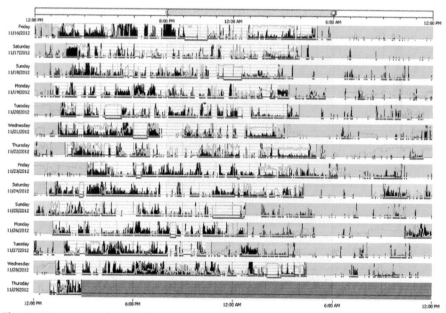

Fig. 1. Wrist actigraphy data from a patient with DSWPD. Each row of data presents a 24-hour time interval, with this example starting from 12 PM, through 12 AM (*middle of the graph*), through the following 12 PM. Yellow data lines represent ambient light exposure. Black vertical columns represent amount of physical activity as measured in 1-minute intervals. The horizontal light-blue, shaded areas represent time intervals in which the patient reported being in bed trying to sleep.

Additional Measures to Support Diagnosis

Objective measures of circadian phase, the most reliable of which is the dim light melatonin onset (DLMO),[13] are currently listed as options, rather than guidelines or standards, as there is not currently evidence to support routinely recommending their use in clinical practice settings.[9] Although DLMO is often used in research settings to provide objective markers of an individual's circadian phase, and has shown to have week-to-week stability in patients with DSWPD,[12] the cost and burden of collecting DLMO would be prohibitive in many clinical settings.[14] As additional research is conducted, utilization of DLMO in assessment and treatment of DSWPD and ASWPD may help to assist with differential diagnosis or refinement of treatment recommendations. **Fig. 2** displays the DLMO profile of an individual without a sleep complaint compared with the DLMO profile of a prototypical patient with DSWPD.

The morningness-eveningness questionnaire (MEQ) has also been listed as an option for assessment of DSWPD and ASWPD.[9] The MEQ[15] provides an estimate of when an individual prefers to engage in activity, such as work, and when the individual prefers to sleep and wake. This questionnaire can be used to assess a continuum of morning preference (morningness) to evening preference (eveningness) or can be used to classify individuals into the chronotypes of morning type ("lark"), neutral type, or evening type ("night owl"). Chronotype has been found to correlate with markers of circadian phase; thus, administration of this questionnaire may be helpful in estimating an individual's circadian phase and supporting diagnosis. However, the MEQ asks about preferences, not current behaviors, so an individual could be classified as an evening or morning chronotype, yet may be functioning with a normal sleep-wake schedule and not have a delayed or advanced circadian system. Thus, this

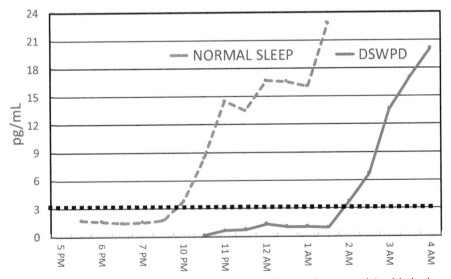

Fig. 2. Salivary DLMO data comparing an individual without a sleep complaint (*dashed orange line*) with a patient with DSWPD (*solid blue line*). The interpolated clock time where the melatonin values cross a threshold (3 pg/mL in this example) is reported as the time of DLMO.

questionnaire should not be used as the sole determinant of whether an individual meets the criteria for DSWPD or ASWPD. Alternative chronotype assessment questionnaires exist for adults[16] and children.[17]

COMORBIDITIES
Insomnia

Insomnia may co-occur with DSWPD.[5,6,18] Conditioned arousal, in which the bed becomes a conditioned stimulus for arousal, may develop from spending long periods in bed when attempting to sleep during times that are societally normative. This conditioned arousal could then lead to comorbid insomnia that may need to be treated in addition to the circadian rhythm disorder.

Other Psychiatric Diagnoses

DSWPD is highly comorbid with a variety of psychiatric diagnoses, which may impact assessment and treatment. Kripke and colleagues[19] found that 44% of their sample with DSWPD reported having attended psychotherapy, compared with 21% of controls. Delayed sleep-wake times have been associated with bipolar diagnoses.[20] A high proportion of those with severe obsessive-compulsive disorder have been found to have DSWPD.[21]

Reid and colleagues[22] found that among a sample of those with DSWPD and those who were evening chronotypes (not diagnosed with DSWPD), more than one-third of those with DSWPD had a history of major depressive disorder and substance use disorders. Interestingly, those who were evening chronotypes had higher rates of these and other psychiatric disorders as diagnosed by the Structured Clinical Interview for the DSM, indicating that these relationships may be related to chronotype rather than DSWPD. Although DSWPD is typically discussed as an intrinsic sleep disorder, evening chronotype might contribute to behavioral delays that might maintain or exacerbate the disorder.

There has been a dearth of research examining comorbidities accompanying ASWPD.

TREATMENTS FOR DELAYED SLEEP-WAKE PHASE DISORDER AND ADVANCED SLEEP-WAKE PHASE DISORDER
Chronotherapy

Chronotherapy for delayed sleep-wake phase disorder
Chronotherapy was created by Czeisler and colleagues[23] as a way to shift the sleep-wake cycle of an individual with DSWPD. It was postulated that individuals with DSWPD can entrain their rhythms and maintain a consistent sleep-wake schedule, albeit delayed; however, these individuals cannot advance their rhythms. Thus, to shift their sleep-wake schedule, those with DSWPD would need to progressively delay their sleep period until reaching their desired sleep-wake schedule. Chronotherapy sets an individual on a 27-hour sleep-wake schedule, with prescribed bedtime being 3 hours later each day. Once the desired sleep schedule has been reached, the new bedtime and wake time are maintained. Other variants of scheduling also have been used (eg, 2-hour delays, twice per week).[24]

There have been no randomized controlled trials assessing the efficacy of chronotherapy for DSWPD. Evidence for the use of this therapy is limited to case studies, which have shown mixed results.[23–25] Given the lack of controlled trials, it is difficult to draw conclusions regarding the effectiveness of this intervention, or for whom the intervention might be most successful. It could be postulated that this method is more successful for those with longer circadian periods (eg, 24.7 hours), given how large the required delays are, rather than those with an average period (~24.2 hours[26,27]). In addition, an individual must have a flexible schedule when engaging in this therapy, given that for a period of time, the individual's sleep period will be during the day and wake period during the night.

Chronotherapy for advanced sleep-wake phase disorder

Evidence for the use of phase advance chronotherapy as the sole treatment for ASWPD is minimal. One case study documented an individual with ASWPD who was put to bed 3 hours earlier every 2 days until the goal bedtime of 11:00 PM was reached.[28] Follow-up 5 months posttreatment demonstrated that this individual was able to maintain his bedtime of 11:00 PM and wake time of 7:00 AM Of note, the individual presented within the case study was also found to have mild obstructive sleep apnea (OSA) on baseline polysomnography. The case study did not detail whether OSA was treated, which would be pertinent to fully comprehend treatment effects. Further research is necessary to support the use of phase advance chronotherapy.

Sleep Scheduling

In both DSWPD and ASWPD, sleep scheduling is inherent in chronotherapy and is used in concert with bright light therapy and treatment with melatonin. Sleep scheduling, which consists of prescribing bedtimes and wake times, helps to entrain an individual's circadian rhythm and consistently build homeostatic drive for sleep. In addition, sleep scheduling helps to ensure an individual can receive other components of treatment at appropriate times. For instance, maintaining a consistent wake-up time will help to ensure an individual with DSWPD is able to use morning bright light therapy at the appropriate time.

Phototherapy

Before the 1980s, it was thought that human circadian rhythms were entrained by zeitgebers (time cues) such as social interactions, feeding schedules, and behavioral sleep-wake cycles, rather than light-dark cycles, as in other living organisms. Czeisler and colleagues[29] investigated the effect of light and dark cycles in a healthy 66-year-old woman under a constant routine protocol. Early evening artificial light exposure (7000–12,000 lux, similar to outdoor ambient light just after dawn) produced a 6-hour phase delay in minimum core body temperature (CBTmin), which demonstrated that light and dark cycles alone could entrain the circadian system. Subsequent studies by Czeisler and his group provided further evidence for this theory,[30,31] and helped to lay the foundation for the development of phototherapy protocols to treat DSWPD and ASWPD. **Fig. 3** displays a simplification of what is called a "phase response curve to light" ("PRC"). Light exposure in the evening hours before routine bedtime through the first two-thirds of the night result in a circadian phase delay, whereas light exposure at the end of the habitual sleep episode through the morning hours results in a circadian phase advance. The "crossover zone" is a time point before which phase delaying occurs and after which phase advancing occurs. This zone is typically found approximately 90 to 120 minutes before habitual wake-up time.

Phototherapy for delayed sleep-wake phase disorder

Bright light exposure synchronizes or entrains the endogenous circadian rhythm, shifts circadian phase,[32] and suppresses nocturnal melatonin release.[33] Bright light differentially impacts the circadian system depending on circadian phase of light administration, and phase response curves have been created to describe the magnitude and direction of circadian phase shift based on timing, duration, and intensity of

CIRCADIAN PHASE SHIFTING FROM BRIGHT LIGHT

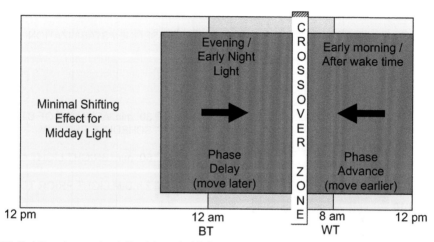

NOTE: Clock times denote only to habitual sleep schedule for sample patient, not to absolute clock time for all

Fig. 3. A simplification of the PRC to light. Depending on the timing of ocular exposure to light relative to circadian phase, the circadian system may shift later ("phase delaying") or earlier ("phase advancing"). BT, bed time; WT, wake time.

light exposure.[34–36] When attempting to phase advance the internal clock, it is important to treat with light after the nadir of core body temperature (CBTmin), which occurs approximately 2 hours before habitual wake time.[37] Studies have used bright white or full-spectrum light (which uses a mixed spectrum of wavelengths, simulating daylight) at 2500 lux for 2 to 3 hours before rise time.[37,38] Other studies have also shown that using blue light (approximately 460 nm) or longer periods of moderate intensity of light are more effective than bright white light in shifting circadian phase.[39]

Bright light therapy is indicated in the treatment of DSWPD; however, the optimal timing, dosing, and duration are unclear.[9] Various phototherapy protocols have been published.[40] Currently, the American Academy of Sleep Medicine (AASM) Clinical Practice Guidelines suggest that clinicians treat children and adolescents with DSWPD with postawakening light therapy.[41] No recommendation for morning light therapy for adults with DSWPD is given in the latest guidelines, likely because strong evidence of optimal administration techniques and treatment benefit is lacking.

Light exposure in the evening or any time before one's CBTmin can theoretically worsen DSWPD, thus avoiding light at night may be recommended as an adjunct to bright light therapy.[42] There is currently insufficient evidence to support avoiding evening light as stand-alone treatment for DSWPD.[41,43]

As there is no "gold-standard" protocol of phototherapy for treatment of any of the circadian rhythm sleep-wake disorders, an example is provided in **Fig. 4** for the treatment of DSWPD, as developed by the senior author (JKW) of this article. The protocol consists of prescribing the patient to stabilizing his or her sleep schedule to the timing usually kept on ad libitum times such as weekends or vacations, then a progressive shift earlier of the sleep schedule by 30 minutes per day. Dim light exposure is prescribed for the 2-hours before bedtime to permit endogenous melatonin release and

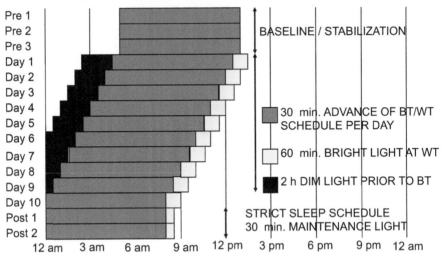

Fig. 4. Phototherapy treatment protocol example for a patient with DSWPD. In this example, the pretreatment delayed sleep schedule was from 5 AM to 1 PM, with a desired, posttreatment sleep schedule from midnight to 8 AM. As described in the text, treatment components include avoidance of bright light exposure for 2 hours before bedtime, moving the sleep schedule earlier 30 minutes per day, and exposure to bright light for 60 minutes following wake-up time. BT, bed time; WT, wake time.

to prevent light exposure when it might worsen the phase delay. Artificial bright light or sunlight exposure is prescribed for 60 minutes following each wake-up time, to phase advance the circadian system. After reaching the desired sleep timing, strict adherence to the sleep schedule is recommended, along with a maintenance dose of 30 minutes of bright light following wake-up time to maintain entrainment at this earlier clock time.

Phototherapy for advanced sleep-wake phase disorder

Data are limited regarding the treatment of ASWPD with phototherapy. Multiple studies have shown a successful delay in circadian phase with exposure to evening bright light in elderly patients; however, patients reported difficulty tolerating the light, which resulted in poor adherence.[44,45] Palmer and colleagues[46] found that patients exposed to dim light at night were more compliant and experienced similar symptomatic benefit than those treated with a higher intensity light therapy. Munch and colleagues[47] demonstrated that evening light improved subjective alertness, increased wake alpha electroencephalogram activity, and increased rapid eye movement latency in older patients with "difficulty sleeping," suggesting that light therapy can be beneficial for sleepiness in the early evening.

Patients with ASWPD who use phototherapy with dim light rather than bright light generally report reasonable adherence, limited side effects, and high satisfaction in terms of symptom improvement and affordability of treatment.[46] In light of this, current

AASM Clinical Practice Guidelines suggest that clinicians treat adults with evening light phototherapy despite very low quality evidence currently available. Due to lack of evidence, strategic avoidance of light in these patients is not recommended.[41]

Side effects
There are minimal side effects associated with phototherapy. Hypomania has been described as a potential adverse effect of light therapy; however, it is still often used safely in mood disorders, including bipolar disorder, as long as the patient is closely monitored by a health care professional.[48,49] Eyestrain, nausea, agitation, and headaches are other reported mild side effects that usually spontaneously resolve.[50]

Melatonin Administration

Melatonin is a hormone made primarily by the pineal gland. Endogenous melatonin impacts circadian rhythms and sleep, temperature regulation, reproductive cycles, mood, tumor growth, and aging.[51] Melatonin supplementation follows a phase response curve nearly inverse to what is seen with bright light therapy.[33,52] Exogenous melatonin also has a hypnotic effect, without an apparent dose-response function, and limited to administration during the biological day when endogenous melatonin is absent.[53]

Melatonin for delayed sleep-wake phase disorder
In DSWPD, melatonin is administered in the evening to entrain the endogenous circadian rhythm and promote sleep. Studies have demonstrated the phase-advancing effects of 0.3 to 5.0 mg of melatonin.[54,55] Timing of melatonin administration impacts the magnitude of phase advance, whereas higher doses of melatonin do not,[56] indicating that there may not be a dose-response effect of melatonin treatment. Studies have demonstrated that administering melatonin in the late afternoon or early evening (some protocols involved administration at 5 or fewer hours before average bedtime; other studies explored melatonin dosing 5 hours before DLMO) in patients with DSWPD advances rhythms.[54,55]

Unfortunately, patients may experience a relapse of symptoms if melatonin administration is stopped.[54–56] Timing of symptom recurrence has been associated with severity of pretreatment circadian delay.[55]

Overall, the evidence for melatonin use in DSWPD is weak and does not demonstrate consistent clinical benefit among patients. Despite this, the AASM suggests that adults and children with DSWPD are treated with strategically timed melatonin (before DLMO, typically between 7 and 9 PM), rather than no treatment at all.[41] This is likely because melatonin has a good safety profile and potential benefits of treatment, even if subtle, outweigh the risks. When considering treatment course, it is reasonable to treat patients with a more severe delay in circadian phase with a longer course of melatonin to provide a more sustained treatment response.

Melatonin for advanced sleep-wake phase disorder
Melatonin administration in the morning can delay circadian rhythms in patients without sleep disorders.[52] Less is known about the efficacy of timed melatonin in patients with ASWPD. Although properly timed melatonin may theoretically improve symptoms of ASWPD, there is no direct evidence demonstrating the efficacy of this intervention.[57] In addition, melatonin has a soporific effect[58]; thus, administration of melatonin in the morning may lead to difficulty with remaining awake, making it more difficult to adhere to scheduled sleep and wake times. Given this, the AASM

does not currently recommend morning administration of supplemental melatonin or melatonin agonists to treat ASWPD.[41]

Side effects

At low doses (0.5 mg–5.0 mg), reported side effects of melatonin, including headache, nausea, dizziness, and drowsiness, tend to be mild and usually do not prompt patients to stop treatment.[59] Some patients may experience increased depressive symptoms.[60] Rare case reports also have associated exogenous melatonin administration with impaired glucose tolerance and alopecia areata.[41,61] Interactions between supplemental melatonin and vitamin K still need to be explored; therefore, melatonin should be used with caution in patients on warfarin.[62] Caution also should be taken in patients with epilepsy. At higher doses, melatonin has a hypnotic effect when taken during the day.[63]

It also has been suggested that exogenous melatonin may affect reproductive development and growth hormone regulation; however, studies have not found evidence of these changes in children on long-term supplemental melatonin.[64–66] Although it is unlikely that short-term use has a negative impact in these systems, one should consider these interactions before prescribing melatonin in children and adolescents.

Long-term safety data are sparse, but suggest extremely low risk of adverse effects in patients taking continuous melatonin. Due to limited data, women who are pregnant or breast feeding should avoid taking supplemental melatonin.[67] Of note, melatonin is considered a "dietary supplement" rather than a pharmaceutical drug. There is heterogeneity in melatonin formulations between brands and no absolute guidelines exist regarding the manufacturing of these supplements. Based on the data available, there is no evidence of adverse effects of melatonin with short-term use, defined as days to weeks.[59]

Hypnotics

Delayed sleep-wake phase disorder

There is little evidence for the use of hypnotics, such as benzodiazepines and nonbenzodiazepine benzodiazepine receptor agonists (or "BZRAs" such as zolpidem, zaleplon, eszopiclone), to treat DSWPD. Of the studies available, most studied the use of hypnotics alongside chronotherapy. In one study, triazolam, a short-acting benzodiazepine, helped maintain the results of chronotherapy in a small group of patients.[68]

Advanced sleep-wake phase disorder

To our knowledge, there are no studies that have evaluated the use of hypnotics in ASWPD.

Side effects

Clinicians should hesitate before prescribing sedative hypnotics. Many medications used to facilitate sleep have been linked to adverse drug events, hospitalizations, and increased mortality in older patients, and have even been considered "potentially inappropriate medications" by the American Geriatrics Society (AGS).[69] Benzodiazepines specifically are metabolized slowly in the geriatric population and increase the risk of cognitive impairment, falls, delirium, fractures, and motor vehicle accidents. Although the nonbenzodiazepine benzodiazepine receptor agonists (such as zolpidem, zaleplon, and eszopiclone) have a shorter half-life and are believed to be safer, the AGS recommends limiting their use to less than 90 days because of a similar side-effect profile as benzodiazepines. It is also recommended to avoid antihistamines because of significant side effects, including cognitive impairment, anticholinergic effects, and daytime sleepiness.[70] Hypnotic medications also have the potential for abuse and should be avoided in patients at high risk for addiction.

Cognitive-Behavioral Therapy

Components of cognitive-behavioral therapies (eg, sleep hygiene, stimulus control, motivational interviewing, relaxation strategies, cognitive therapy) may be useful when treating those with DSWPD and ASWPD. As noted previously, individuals with circadian rhythm disorders may have comorbid insomnia. These individuals may benefit from receiving cognitive-behavioral therapy for insomnia along with treatment for their circadian rhythm disturbance. In addition, treating circadian rhythm sleep disorders requires significant behavior change, leading some investigators to hypothesize that cognitive-behavioral therapy may be necessary to assist patients in maintaining treatment gains.[71,72] Those with DSWPD also may experience cognitive processes[73] and demonstrate low readiness to change or low self-efficacy[74] that would benefit from treatment with cognitive-behavioral therapies. Cognitive-behavioral therapy has been added to bright light therapy for those with DSWPD, with good results; however, the extent to which cognitive-behavioral therapy improves treatment above and beyond bright light therapy alone remains to be seen.[5,71]

To our knowledge, there have been no studies examining cognitive-behavioral therapy as an adjunct to bright light therapy in ASWPD.

Treatment Maintenance

To maintain treatment gains, patients need to continue using sleep scheduling, and often may benefit from continued use of melatonin and/or bright light therapy, given that individuals who stop treatment typically experience symptom relapse.[55] More studies are needed to further delineate factors that play a role in duration of treatment response and maintenance of treatment gains when using melatonin and phototherapy.

CONCLUSIONS

Most research studies examining treatments for DSWPD and ASWPD have focused on phototherapy and melatonin administration. Some support exists for the use of chronotherapy; however, there are no randomized controlled trials to support its use. Although this treatment may be beneficial for some, those who engage in this therapy must be able to devote a significant amount of time to treatment, given the prescribed progressively delayed sleep schedule.

More robust studies are needed to determine the optimal prescriptions for timing and intensity of bright light therapy for patients with circadian rhythm disorders. Light therapy is commonly used in clinical practice because many existing studies suggest its efficacy and limited alternative treatments. Similarly, appropriately timed melatonin appears to be a safe option for treatment of circadian rhythm disorders and has slightly more evidence for clinical improvement; however, more data are needed to make strong recommendations for these conditions. Components of cognitive-behavioral therapy also may improve adherence to treatments or improve the ability to maintain treatment gains; however, more research is necessary to support this statement.

Summary and Future Directions

As relatively young health care specialties, sleep medicine and behavioral sleep medicine have many challenges ahead with respect to the circadian rhythm sleep-wake disorders. One of the biggest challenges will be consideration of objective measures of circadian phase position in patients with DSWPD and ASWPD. As it currently stands, the ICSD-3 requires neither objective measurement of circadian phase nor confirmation of a mismatch between circadian phase and the desired sleep schedule. For the first few decades of human circadian rhythms research, circadian phase assessment used the measurement of core body temperature as the gold standard (eg, Refs.[75,76]). Controversy surrounded so-called "demasking" techniques, which promised to allow for measurement of circadian phase from ambulatory core temperature measurement.[77] Accurate data collection required a host of expensive, labor-intensive, intrusive methods, such as keeping the participant awake for 30+ hours while on bedrest: the so-called "constant routine" protocol.[78] Gradually, core body temperature was replaced with circadian phase measurement via frequent blood sampling to assay for melatonin levels during dim light conditions, either limited to capturing its pre–sleep-onset ("DLMO", eg, Ref.[13]) or the entire nocturnal melatonin profile.[75,79] Higher cost-effectiveness and decreased burden have been realized with DLMO estimation via saliva samples instead of blood, and protocols have been tested to allow participants to collect these at home.[80,81]

Several scenarios might hasten the adoption of salivary DLMO assessment in these patients. First, it might be possible to improve the accuracy of diagnosis in these patients, particularly in the complicated differential diagnosis of DSWPD from a variety of conditions leading to sleep-onset insomnia,[82] and distinguishing ASWPD from insomnia with early morning awakening (EMA), or major depression with EMA. The need for this is highlighted by recent data finding that 43% of individuals meeting ICSD-2 criteria for DSWPD did not have the anticipated delay in DLMO, indicating that reliance on self-report alone may lead to an improper diagnosis.[83] Second, advancing or delaying circadian phase, via delivery of timed bright light exposure (phototherapy) and/or using oral melatonin, could be more potent if circadian phase was known. For example, there are substantial differences in the amount of phase advance that can be delivered from single pulses of bright light depending on relatively small differences in circadian phase.[32,34] Finally, assessment of circadian phase would be desirable to confirm treatment outcome, or to suggest suboptimal adherence in treatment failures.

Optimization of the manipulation of circadian phase via melatonin is another area ripe for improvement. Using melatonin to phase advance a patient with DSWPD requires rigid adherence to timed administration of oral melatonin,[84] involves administration many hours before bedtime risking suboptimal alertness during the latter portion of the waking day (via suppression of circadian alerting), and risks return of symptoms on melatonin discontinuation.[54] Perhaps worse is the need to awaken a patient with ASWPD toward the end of the sleep episode to ingest melatonin during the optimal phase-delay region of the PRC to melatonin, and the paucity of research to support efficacy and safety of melatonin in treating ASWPD.[57] Simpler, or better-timed pharmacologic interventions are desirable.

Shifting circadian phase with timed bright light is also a complicated, demanding treatment option. Advancing a patient with DSWPD requires access to a bright light source for perhaps an hour each morning after awakening, which can conflict with preparations and travel to school, work, or other daily activities. Also, the time to deliver light to achieve maximal phase advance or phase delay, according to the phase response curve for light, is during the middle third (to phase advance) or last third (to phase delay) of the sleep episode. Patients with a sleep disorder should not be required to wake up to engage in a treatment, compounding rather than alleviating their sleep loss. Although there were early failures to shift circadian phase with light exposure delivered to sleeping patients, more recent work suggests this may be possible.[85]

A final area quite in need of more research pertains to exposure to bright light in the presleep period, with particular focus on light in the blue to green wavelength range (eg, 470–525 nm) to which the circadian system is most sensitive.[86] Early work[87] in this area has suggested such light exposure could delay circadian phase and sleep onset, but by amounts statistically but likely not clinically meaningful. There also have been challenges to that experiment pointing to various unrepresentative study conditions that would not generalize to the population.[88] Newer research has suggested that there may be gender differences in physiologic response to presleep blue-enriched light exposure, and that within male individuals the effects on subsequent sleep may be neutral to actually beneficial, correlating with the subjective perception of the brightness of the light.[89] Clearly the evidence-based practice of sleep medicine or behavioral sleep medicine requires caution before making any strong recommendations based on these scant, and sometimes paradoxic findings about the use (or avoidance) of light exposure before bedtime.

REFERENCES

1. Weitzman ED, Czeisler CA, Coleman RM, et al. Delayed sleep phase syndrome. A chronobiological disorder with sleep-onset insomnia. Arch Gen Psychiatry 1981;38(7):737–46.
2. Kamei R, Hughes L, Miles L, et al. Advanced-sleep phase syndrome studied in a time isolation facility. Chronobiologia 1979;6:115.
3. Borbély AA. A two process model of sleep regulation. Hum Neurobiol 1982;1(3): 195–204.
4. Wyatt JK. Delayed sleep phase syndrome: pathophysiology and treatment options. Sleep 2004;27(6):1195–203.
5. Gradisar M, Dohnt H, Gardner G, et al. A randomized controlled trial of cognitive-behavior therapy plus bright light therapy for adolescent delayed sleep phase disorder. Sleep 2011;34(12):1671–80.
6. Cvengros JA, Wyatt JK. Circadian rhythm disorders. Sleep Med Clin 2009;4(4): 495–505.
7. American Academy of Sleep Medicine. International classification of sleep disorders. 3rd edition. Darien (IL): American Academy of Sleep Medicine; 2014.
8. American Psychiatric Association. Diagnostic and statistical manual of mental disorders: DSM-5. Arlington (VA): American Psychiatric Publishing; 2013.
9. Morgenthaler TI, Lee-Chiong T, Alessi C, et al. Practice parameters for the clinical evaluation and treatment of circadian rhythm sleep disorders. An American Academy of Sleep Medicine report. Sleep 2007;30(11):1445–59.
10. Carney CE, Buysse DJ, Ancoli-Israel S, et al. The consensus sleep diary: standardizing prospective sleep self-monitoring. Sleep 2012;35(2):287–302.
11. Morgenthaler T, Alessi C, Friedman L, et al. Practice parameters for the use of actigraphy in the assessment of sleep and sleep disorders: an update for 2007. Sleep 2007;30(4):519–29.
12. Wyatt JK, Stepanski EJ, Kirkby J. Circadian phase in delayed sleep phase syndrome: predictors and temporal stability across multiple assessments. Sleep 2006;29(8):1075–80.
13. Lewy AJ, Sack RL. The dim light melatonin onset as a marker for circadian phase position. Chronobiol Int 1989;6(1):93–102.
14. Keijzer H, Smits MG, Duffy JF, et al. Why the dim light melatonin onset (DLMO) should be measured before treatment of patients with circadian rhythm sleep disorders. Sleep Med Rev 2014;18(4):333–9.

15. Horne JA, Ostberg O. A self-assessment questionnaire to determine morningness-eveningness in human circadian rhythms. Int J Chronobiol 1976; 4(2):97–110.
16. Roenneberg T, Wirz-Justice A, Merrow M. Life between clocks: daily temporal patterns of human chronotypes. J Biol Rhythms 2003;18(1):80–90.
17. Werner H, Lebourgeois MK, Geiger A, et al. Assessment of chronotype in four- to eleven-year-old children: reliability and validity of the Children's Chronotype Questionnaire (CCTQ). Chronobiol Int 2009;26(5):992–1014.
18. Sivertsen B, Pallesen S, Stormark KM, et al. Delayed sleep phase syndrome in adolescents: prevalence and correlates in a large population based study. BMC Public Health 2013;13:1163.
19. Kripke DF, Rex KM, Ancoli-Israel S, et al. Delayed sleep phase cases and controls. J Circadian Rhythms 2008;6:6.
20. Robillard R, Naismith SL, Rogers NL, et al. Delayed sleep phase in young people with unipolar or bipolar affective disorders. J Affect Disord 2013;145(2):260–3.
21. Turner J, Drummond LM, Mukhopadhyay S, et al. A prospective study of delayed sleep phase syndrome in patients with severe resistant obsessive-compulsive disorder. World Psychiatry 2007;6(2):108–11.
22. Reid KJ, Jaksa AA, Eisengart JB, et al. Systematic evaluation of Axis-I DSM diagnoses in delayed sleep phase disorder and evening-type circadian preference. Sleep Med 2012;13(9):1171–7.
23. Czeisler CA, Richardson GS, Coleman RM, et al. Chronotherapy: resetting the circadian clocks of patients with delayed sleep phase insomnia. Sleep 1981; 4(1):1–21.
24. Alvarez B, Dahlitz MJ, Vignau J, et al. The delayed sleep phase syndrome: clinical and investigative findings in 14 subjects. J Neurol Neurosurg Psychiatry 1992;55(8):665–70.
25. Ito A, Ando K, Hayakawa T, et al. Long-term course of adult patients with delayed sleep phase syndrome. Jpn J Psychiatry Neurol 1993;47(3):563–7.
26. Burgess HJ, Eastman CI. Human tau in an ultradian light-dark cycle. J Biol Rhythms 2008;23(4):374–6.
27. Czeisler CA, Duffy JF, Shanahan TL, et al. Stability, precision, and near-24-hour period of the human circadian pacemaker. Science 1999;284(5423):2177–81.
28. Moldofsky H, Musisi S, Phillipson EA. Treatment of a case of advanced sleep phase syndrome by phase advance chronotherapy. Sleep 1986;9(1):61–5.
29. Czeisler CA, Allan JS, Strogatz SH, et al. Bright light resets the human circadian pacemaker independent of the timing of the sleep-wake cycle. Science 1986; 233(4764):667–71.
30. Strogatz SH, Kronauer RE, Czeisler CA. Circadian regulation dominates homeostatic control of sleep length and prior wake length in humans. Sleep 1986;9(2): 353–64.
31. Czeisler CA, Kronauer RE, Allan JS, et al. Bright light induction of strong (type 0) resetting of the human circadian pacemaker. Science 1989;244(4910):1328–33.
32. St Hilaire MA, Gooley JJ, Khalsa SB, et al. Human phase response curve to a 1 h pulse of bright white light. J Physiol 2012;590(Pt 13):3035–45.
33. Lewy AJ, Wehr TA, Goodwin FK, et al. Light suppresses melatonin secretion in humans. Science 1980;210:1267–9.
34. Khalsa SB, Jewett ME, Cajochen C, et al. A phase response curve to single bright light pulses in human subjects. J Physiol 2003;549(Pt 3):945–52.
35. Honma K, Honma S. A human phase response curve for bright light pulses. Jpn J Psychiatry Neurol 1988;42(1):167–8.

36. Boivin DB, Duffy JF, Kronauer RE, et al. Dose-response relationships for resetting of human circadian clock by light. Nature 1996;379(6565):540–2.
37. Rosenthal NE, Joseph-Vanderpool JR, Levendosky AA, et al. Phase-shifting effects of bright morning light as treatment for delayed sleep phase syndrome. Sleep 1990;13(4):354–61.
38. Cole RJ, Smith JS, Alcala YC, et al. Bright-light mask treatment of delayed sleep phase syndrome. J Biol Rhythms 2002;17(1):89–101.
39. Dewan K, Benloucif S, Reid K, et al. Light-induced changes of the circadian clock of humans: increasing duration is more effective than increasing light intensity. Sleep 2011;34(5):593–9.
40. Wyatt JK. Circadian rhythm sleep disorders in children and adolescents. Sleep Med Clin 2007;2(3):387–96.
41. Auger RR, Burgess HJ, Emens JS, et al. Clinical practice guideline for the treatment of intrinsic Circadian Rhythm sleep-wake disorders: advanced sleep-wake phase disorder (ASWPD), delayed sleep-wake phase disorder (DSWPD), non-24-hour sleep-wake rhythm disorder (N24SWD), and irregular sleep-wake rhythm disorder (ISWRD). An update for 2015: An American Academy of Sleep Medicine Clinical Practice Guideline. J Clin Sleep Med 2015;11(10):1199–236.
42. Burkhart K, Phelps JR. Amber lenses to block blue light and improve sleep: a randomized trial. Chronobiol Int 2009;26(8):1602–12.
43. Auger RR, Burgess HJ, Dierkhising RA, et al. Light exposure among adolescents with delayed sleep phase disorder: a prospective cohort study. Chronobiol Int 2011;28(10):911–20.
44. Campbell SS, Murphy PJ, van den Heuvel CJ, et al. Etiology and treatment of intrinsic circadian rhythm sleep disorders. Sleep Med Rev 1999;3(3):179–200.
45. Suhner AG, Murphy PJ, Campbell SS. Failure of timed bright light exposure to alleviate age-related sleep maintenance insomnia. J Am Geriatr Soc 2002; 50(4):617–23.
46. Palmer CR, Kripke DF, Savage HC Jr, et al. Efficacy of enhanced evening light for advanced sleep phase syndrome. Behav Sleep Med 2003;1(4):213–26.
47. Munch M, Scheuermaier KD, Zhang R, et al. Effects on subjective and objective alertness and sleep in response to evening light exposure in older subjects. Behav Brain Res 2011;224(2):272–8.
48. Dauphinais DR, Rosenthal JZ, Terman M, et al. Controlled trial of safety and efficacy of bright light therapy vs. negative air ions in patients with bipolar depression. Psychiatry Res 2012;196(1):57–61.
49. Tuunainen A, Kripke DF, Endo T. Light therapy for non-seasonal depression. Cochrane Database Syst Rev 2004;(2):CD004050.
50. Meesters Y, van Houwelingen CA. Rapid mood swings after unmonitored light exposure. Am J Psychiatry 1998;155(2):306.
51. Brzezinski A. Melatonin in humans. N Engl J Med 1997;336(3):186–95.
52. Lewy AJ, Bauer VK, Ahmed S, et al. The human phase response curve (PRC) to melatonin is about 12 hours out of phase with the PRC to light. Chronobiol Int 1998;15(1):71–83.
53. Wyatt JK, Dijk DJ, Ritz-de Cecco A, et al. Sleep-facilitating effect of exogenous melatonin in healthy young men and women is circadian-phase dependent. Sleep 2006;29(5):609–18.
54. Dahlitz M, Alvarez B, Vignau J, et al. Delayed sleep phase syndrome response to melatonin. Lancet 1991;337(8750):1121–4.

55. Dagan Y, Yovel I, Hallis D, et al. Evaluating the role of melatonin in the long-term treatment of delayed sleep phase syndrome (DSPS). Chronobiol Int 1998;15(2): 181–90.

56. Mundey K, Benloucif S, Harsanyi K, et al. Phase-dependent treatment of delayed sleep phase syndrome with melatonin. Sleep 2005;28(10):1271–8.

57. Zee PC. Melatonin for the treatment of advanced sleep phase disorder. Sleep 2008;31(7):923.

58. van den Heuvel CJ, Ferguson SA, Macchi MM, et al. Comment on 'Melatonin as a hypnotic: pro'. Sleep Med Rev 2005;9(1):67–8 [discussion: 69–70].

59. Buscemi N, Vandermeer B, Pandya R, et al. Melatonin for treatment of sleep disorders. Evidence report/Technology assessment No. 108. (Prepared by the University of Alberta Evidence-based Practice Center, under Contract No. 290-02-0023.) AHRQ Publication No. 05-E002-2. Rockville, MD 2004 2004.

60. Carman JS, Post RM, Buswell R, et al. Negative effects of melatonin on depression. Am J Psychiatry 1976;133(10):1181–6.

61. Rubio-Sastre P, Scheer FA, Gomez-Abellan P, et al. Acute melatonin administration in humans impairs glucose tolerance in both the morning and evening. Sleep 2014;37(10):1715–9.

62. Herxheimer A, Petrie KJ. Melatonin for the prevention and treatment of jet lag. Cochrane Database Syst Rev 2002;(2):CD001520.

63. van den Heuvel CJ, Ferguson SA, Macchi MM, et al. Melatonin as a hypnotic: con. Sleep Med Rev 2005;9(1):71–80.

64. Valcavi R, Zini M, Maestroni GJ, et al. Melatonin stimulates growth hormone secretion through pathways other than the growth hormone-releasing hormone. Clin Endocrinol (Oxf) 1993;39(2):193–9.

65. Luboshitzky R, Shen-Orr Z, Nave R, et al. Melatonin administration alters semen quality in healthy men. J Androl 2002;23(4):572–8.

66. van Geijlswijk IM, Mol RH, Egberts TC, et al. Evaluation of sleep, puberty and mental health in children with long-term melatonin treatment for chronic idiopathic childhood sleep onset insomnia. Psychopharmacology (Berl) 2011;216(1): 111–20.

67. Andersen LP, Gogenur I, Rosenberg J, et al. The safety of melatonin in humans. Clin Drug Investig 2016;36(3):169–75.

68. Ohta T, Iwata T, Kayukawa Y, et al. Daily activity and persistent sleep-wake schedule disorders. Prog Neuropsychopharmacol Biol Psychiatry 1992;16(4): 529–37.

69. By the American Geriatrics Society Beers Criteria Update Expert Panel. American Geriatrics Society 2015 updated Beers criteria for potentially inappropriate medication use in older adults. J Am Geriatr Soc 2015;63(11):2227–46.

70. Deschenes CL, McCurry SM. Current treatments for sleep disturbances in individuals with dementia. Curr Psychiatry Rep 2009;11(1):20–6.

71. Danielsson K, Jansson-Frojmark M, Broman JE, et al. Cognitive behavioral therapy as an adjunct treatment to light therapy for delayed sleep phase disorder in young adults: a randomized controlled feasibility study. Behav Sleep Med 2016;14(2):212–32.

72. Lack LC, Wright HR. Clinical management of delayed sleep phase disorder. Behav Sleep Med 2007;5(1):57–76.

73. Richardson C, Micic G, Cain N, et al. Cognitive performance in adolescents with delayed sleep-wake phase disorder: treatment effects and a comparison with good sleepers. J Adolesc 2018;65:72–84.

74. Micic G, Richardson C, Cain N, et al. Readiness to change and commitment as predictors of therapy compliance in adolescents with delayed sleep-wake phase disorder. Sleep Med 2018;55:48–55.
75. Shanahan TL, Czeisler CA. Light exposure induces equivalent phase shifts of the endogenous circadian rhythms of circulating plasma melatonin and core body temperature in men. J Clin Endocrinol Metab 1991;73(2):227–35.
76. Czeisler CA, Weitzman E, Moore-Ede MC, et al. Human sleep: its duration and organization depend on its circadian phase. Science 1980;210(4475):1264–7.
77. Klerman EB, Lee Y, Czeisler CA, et al. Linear demasking techniques are unreliable for estimating the circadian phase of ambulatory temperature data. J Biol Rhythms 1999;14(4):260–74.
78. Duffy JF, Dijk DJ. Getting through to circadian oscillators: why use constant routines? J Biol Rhythms 2002;17(1):4–13.
79. Brown EN, Choe Y, Shanahan TL, et al. A mathematical model of diurnal variations in human plasma melatonin levels. Am J Physiol 1997;272(3 Pt 1):E506–16.
80. Burgess HJ, Wyatt JK, Park M, et al. Home circadian phase assessments with measures of compliance yield accurate dim light melatonin onsets. Sleep 2015; 38(6):889–97.
81. Burgess HJ, Park M, Wyatt JK, et al. Home dim light melatonin onsets with measures of compliance in delayed sleep phase disorder. J Sleep Res 2016;25(3): 314–7.
82. Rahman SA, Kayumov L, Tchmoutina EA, et al. Clinical efficacy of dim light melatonin onset testing in diagnosing delayed sleep phase syndrome. Sleep Med 2009;10(5):549–55.
83. Murray JM, Sletten TL, Magee M, et al. Prevalence of circadian misalignment and its association with depressive symptoms in delayed sleep phase disorder. Sleep 2017;40(1).
84. Burgess HJ, Revell VL, Molina TA, et al. Human phase response curves to three days of daily melatonin: 0.5 mg versus 3.0 mg. JClinEndocrinolMetab 2010;95(7): 3325–31.
85. Zeitzer JM, Fisicaro RA, Ruby NF, et al. Millisecond flashes of light phase delay the human circadian clock during sleep. J Biol Rhythms 2014;29(5):370–6.
86. Wright HR, Lack LC. Effect of light wavelength on suppression and phase delay of the melatonin rhythm. Chronobiol Int 2001;18(5):801–8.
87. Chang AM, Aeschbach D, Duffy JF, et al. Evening use of light-emitting eReaders negatively affects sleep, circadian timing, and next-morning alertness. Proc Natl Acad Sci U S A 2015;112(4):1232–7.
88. Zeitzer JM. Real life trumps laboratory in matters of public health. Proc Natl Acad Sci U S A 2015;112(13):E1513.
89. Chellappa SL, Steiner R, Oelhafen P, et al. Sex differences in light sensitivity impact on brightness perception, vigilant attention and sleep in humans. Sci Rep 2017;7(1):14215.

Non–24-hour Sleep-Wake Rhythm Disorder

Sabra M. Abbott, MD, PhD

KEYWORDS

- Circadian • Free-running • Hypernychthemeral • Nonentrained

KEY POINTS

- Non–24-hour sleep-wake rhythm disorder can be seen in both blind and sighted individuals.
- Blind individuals typically lack light perception, whereas pathophysiology for sighted individuals is more complicated.
- Diagnosis requires obtaining a minimum of 2 weeks (preferably longer) of sleep logs and/or actigraphy.
- Treatment focuses on schedule melatonin/melatonin agonists for blind individuals and enhancement of all zeitgebers (eg, light, melatonin, feeding, and social interactions) for sighted individuals.

INTRODUCTION

The human circadian clock has an average period slightly longer than the 24-hour environmental period, of approximately 24.2 hours.[1] The ability to maintain entrainment with the 24-hour environment requires daily adjustments to the circadian clock, either through exposure to environmental light or other timekeeping signals. In the absence of the ability to either receive or respond appropriately to these signals, there is a population of individuals who exhibit a pattern of daily rhythms that typically are longer than 24 hours, every day waking, eating ,and sleeping slightly later than the day before.

CLINICAL PRESENTATION

Non–24-hour sleep-wake rhythm disorder (N24SWD) previously has been referred to as free-running disorder, nonentrained disorder, and hypernychthemeral syndrome. The first published case of an individual with N24SWD was in 1971, describing a man who had a daily rest-activity rhythm of 26 hours and also observed his measured rhythms of cortisol, core body temperature, and electrolyte excretion.[2]

Disclosure Statement: The author has nothing to disclose.
Department of Neurology, Northwestern University Feinberg School of Medicine, 710 North Lake Shore Drive, Abbott Hall 524, Chicago, IL 60610, USA
E-mail address: sabra.abbott@northwestern.edu

Clinically, individuals with N24SWD present with complaints of excessive daytime sleepiness and/or insomnia, which alternate with periods of relatively normal sleep, reflecting the daily delay of rest-activity rhythms, such that these individuals are progressively sleeping in phase and then out of phase with the light-dark environment. An example sleep-wake diary from an individual with N24SWD is shown in **Fig. 1**.

N24SWD has been described in up to 63% of blind individuals who lack light perception,[3] presumably due to the lack of photic input to the suprachiasmatic nucleus; however, this disorder also can be seen in sighted individuals. In the largest case series of sighted individuals, 57 people were described with N24SWD.[4] Among those individuals, 72% were male, and the majority began to exhibit symptoms in the teens or 20s. Similar to patients with delayed sleep-wake phase disorder (DSWPD), there seems to be a high comorbidity of psychiatric disorders in N24SWD. In Hayakawa and colleagus'[4] case series, 28% of their patients had a premorbid psychiatric disorder prior to developing N24SWD, whereas an additional 25% of their cohort developed symptoms of major depression after the onset of N24SWD symptoms. As detailed in a more recent case series of sighted individuals with N24SWD, many of these patients initially present with sleep-wake patterns consistent with DSWPD, typically with very late bedtimes of 3:00 AM to 6:00 AM. They then progress to exhibiting a more non–24-hour pattern and may alternate between a delayed pattern and a non–24-hour pattern.[5] As a consequence, it often can require monitoring for greater than 1 week to confirm the presence of N24SWD.

Within Hayakawa and colleagus'[4] case series, all individuals underwent actigraphy for at least 10 days, which demonstrated an average period of 24.9 hours (range 24.4–26.5 hours). Sleep duration was longer than average, at 9.3 hours ± 1.3 hours. In addition, approximately half of the individuals studied exhibited jumping behavior, whereby they would have greater delays in their rest-activity patterns when sleeping during the day compared with when sleeping at night (**Fig. 2**). For this reason, prior descriptions of this as a free-running disorder seem inaccurate, because these

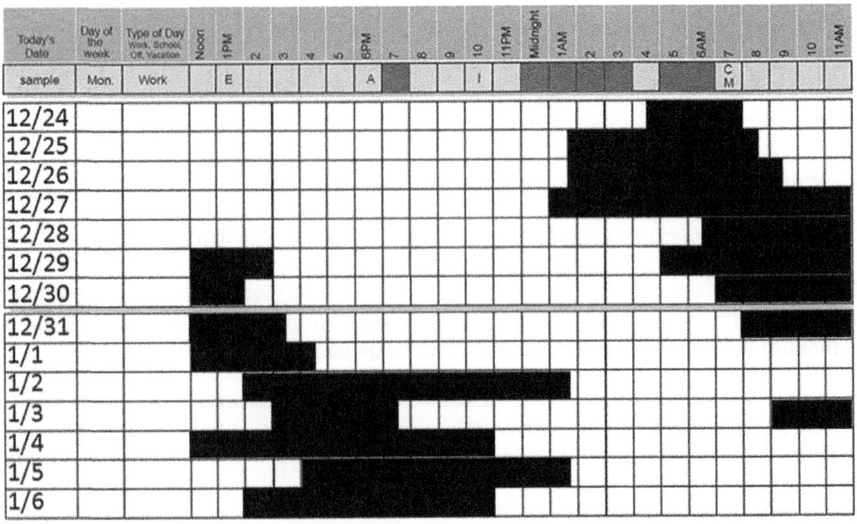

Fig. 1. Example sleep diary from a patient with N24SWD, demonstrating the progressive daily delay of rest-activity patterns. Each line represents 24 hours, with shaded boxes indicating times of sleep.

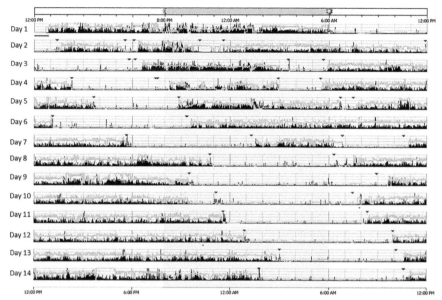

Fig. 2. Actigraphy from a patient with N24SWD demonstrating the variable rate of delay when sleeping at night compared with sleeping during the day. During days 1 to 7, when sleeping during the daytime, the daily rest-activity pattern drifts later much faster than during days 8 to 14, when the patient is sleeping at night. Each line represents 24 hours. Black bars indicate activity, yellow lines indicate light exposure, and blue triangles indicate when the patient went to bed and woke up.

individuals do show signs of being influenced by environmental time cues; however, they are not able to maintain entrainment in response to these cues.

PATHOPHYSIOLOGY OF NON–24-HOUR SLEEP-WAKE RHYTHM DISORDER

Proper alignment of daily rest-activity patterns and other rhythmic behaviors with the environment, a process referred to as *entrainment*, requires the ability to receive and respond to environmental time cues, the strongest of which is light. Exposure to light provides daily adjustments, with light in the evening serving to delay the circadian clock and light in the morning advancing the clock. Because the human circadian clock has an average period of 24.2 hours,[1] without these daily temporal adjustments, there is a potential for a non–24-hour pattern to emerge. The daily environmental light signal is transmitted through melanopsin containing intrinsically photosensitive retinal ganglion cells to the suprachiasmatic nucleus.[6] Thus, is it not surprising that many blind individuals lacking these photoreceptive neural pathways exhibit symptoms of N24SWD. Perhaps more interesting is that 37% to 43% of individuals who lack light perception do not exhibit symptoms of N24SWD.[3,7] Potential explanations for this include having a period that is close enough to 24 hours that significant daily adjustments from light are not required or a strong response to other weaker time cues, such as social interactions and daily patterns of food intake.[8] In the neurology clinic, it is important to consider screening for this disorder in all individuals with impaired retinal ganglion cell-mediated light perception. Examples include patients with bilateral optic neuritis; individuals with Alzheimer disease, which can be associated with retinal ganglion cell degeneration; and patients with severe glaucoma.

There is another category of individuals who report normal visual light perception; however, they exhibit symptoms of N24SWD. The underlying pathophysiology in this case is more complicated and likely multifactorial. Many of these individuals initially present with clinical features of DSWPD but eventually develop a non–24-hour pattern, either naturally or in response to attempts at chronotherapy (deliberately moving behaviors later each day in an attempt to entrain at an earlier phase with respect to the environment). There is evidence in at least some individuals with N24SWD, based on results of a forced desynchrony protocol[9] or fibroblast cultures,[10] that they have a longer circadian period than average, suggesting that they may require stronger entraining signals to maintain a 24-hour rhythm. In addition, a small study has demonstrated that sighted individuals with N24SWD fall asleep closer to their core body temperature nadir compared with controls.[11] Because the core body temperature nadir represents the point at which light switches from causing phase delays to causing phase advances, it is possible that having a sleep-wake pattern with this phase relationship to the environment results in greater exposure to phase-delaying light signals and decreased exposure to phase-advancing signals. There also are case reports describing these individuals as having fewer social interactions and decreased daily light exposure,[5] so the disorder may result from a combination of a pacemaker that is more challenging to entrain, along with mistimed or weak exposure to daily entraining signals. Many of these individuals have been demonstrated to have desynchronization or dampening of some of their biological rhythms, for example, exhibiting robust cortisol and core body temperature rhythms, dampened melatonin rhythms, and a non–24-hour sleep-wake rhythm.[12] Research also is ongoing to determine whether, despite normal visual perception, these individuals may have an impaired ability to respond to circadian light signals.

DIAGNOSIS

A diagnosis of N24SWD depends primarily on documenting a non–24-hour pattern of rest-activity. This is best documented with sleep logs and/or actigraphy monitoring for a minimum of 14 days.[13] Because individuals can fluctuate through times of relative entrainment and times of daily drifting, however, as shown in **Fig. 3**, it can be helpful to obtain records for longer than 2 weeks. Additional testing of phase markers, such as the timing of dim light melatonin onset or the rhythm of the melatonin urinary metabolite 6-sulfatoxymelatonin, also can be useful. In this instance, samples should be obtained 2 weeks to 4 weeks apart and demonstrate a nonentrained rhythm. Standardized chronotype questionnaires are far less useful with this disorder, because responses may vary significantly, depending on when an individual currently is sleeping in relation to the environment.

In diagnosing N24SWD, it is important to distinguish from DSWPD, in which individuals are awake at night and sleeping during the day but do not exhibit a progressive daily delay of their sleep-wake patterns. In the absence of sleep logs and actigraphy, patients with N24SWD may present with a clinical history concerning for irregular sleep-wake rhythm disorder, given the report of episodes of sleeping both during the day and at night. Actigraphy, however, confirms a single sleep bout with progressive daily delay in N24SWD compared with at least 3 separate bouts of sleep within a 24-hour period for irregular sleep-wake rhythm disorder.

TREATMENT

The appropriate treatment of N24SWD depends on the underlying cause of the disorder, with treatment options much better characterized for blind patients compared

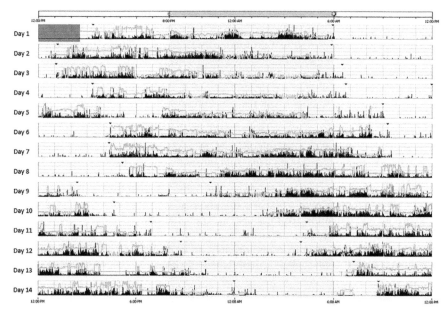

Fig. 3. Actigraphy from a patient with N24SWD. Note that during days 1 to 4 the patient exhibits a fairly stable delayed rest activity pattern, whereas the non–24-hour pattern does not emerge until days 5 to 14. This demonstrates why a single week of actigraphy or sleep logs may not adequately demonstrate the presence of N24SWD. Each line represents 24 hours. Black bars indicate activity, yellow lines indicate light exposure, and blue triangles indicate when the patient went to bed and woke up.

with sighted individuals. Whether blind or sighted, treatment of all individuals focuses on the use of melatonin, both for its circadian resetting properties and its sedating properties.

In blind individuals, the use of melatonin has been well fairly well characterized, although generally in small studies. In 1 of the first case reports of the use of melatonin in a blind individual, administering 5 mg of melatonin, 30 minutes prior to the desired bedtime, resulted in longer total sleep time and decreased daytime napping compared with placebo, although in this patient the core body temperature and cortisol rhythms did not seem to entrain to a 24-hour schedule during melatonin administration.[14] Some individuals, however, do exhibit entrainment of both sleep-wake and cortisol rhythms, as demonstrated by 3 of the 5 blind individuals undergoing a placebo controlled trial of 5 mg of melatonin.[15] Success of entrainment seems to depend in part on the circadian phase at which melatonin was initiated,[16] with studies demonstrating that entrainment does not occur if the phase angle between time of melatonin administration and time of endogenous melatonin onset is greater than 8 hours.[17] Another study demonstrated successful entrainment in 6 of 7 subjects with 10 mg of melatonin, followed by maintenance with 0.5 mg of melatonin.[18] Later studies demonstrated that successful entrainment could be achieved by starting at 0.5 mg and that the initiation phase of 10 mg of melatonin may not be necessary,[19,20] and in some cases lower doses are effective when higher doses are not.[21]

More recently, the Food and Drug Administration approved the use of the melatonin agonist 20 mg for use in the treatment of N24SWD. In randomized placebo-controlled trial administering tasimelteon to 40 blind patients with N24SWD, 20%

showed evidence of entrainment based on the rhythm of urinary 6-sulfatoxymelatonin.[22]

In sighted individuals, treatment protocols are less well defined. There are case reports of administering melatonin (3 mg) at a fixed time, resulting in a 24-hour rhythm of sleep-wake, temperature and cortisol rhythms.[23] In one of the earliest case reports of treatment of a sighted woman with N24SWD, entrainment was achieved through regular 2-hour exposures to bright light therapy immediately after awakening.[24] Another individual was entrained and restored a 24-hour melatonin profile, with a combination of morning bright light for 2 hours, bright light avoidance prior to bedtime, and strict darkness while sleeping.[25] A third individual demonstrated improvement of 24-hour sleep patterns, documented objectively with polysomnography, after 3 hours of morning bright light therapy.[26] Combination therapy, using both light and melatonin has also been attempted, with some initial success, although long-term compliance often is challenging.[27] A more recent article proposed a treatment algorithm using a combination of light and melatonin to entrain sighted patients with N24SWD.[5] Key to that algorithm is waiting to initiate treatment until patients are close to sleeping at their biological bedtime and then trying to use light and melatonin to maintain that timing, rather than using light and melatonin to induce large phase advances or phase delays.

SUMMARY

N24SWD is a rare but clinically important circadian rhythm sleep-wake disorder. It is important for clinicians to be aware of and recognize this disorder not only in their blind patients but also in sighted individuals. Although the non–24-hour pattern is most frequently recognized in the daily rest-activity pattern, it should be recognized that many of these individuals have a desynchronization between their sleep-wake rhythms and other circadian markers, such as melatonin, cortisol, and core body temperature, which can add to the symptom burden in these individuals. As such, it is important to focus on multimodal treatment in these individuals, not only normalizing sleep-wake patterns with melatonin but also focusing on other weaker time cues, such as activity, feeding patterns, and social interactions.

REFERENCES

1. Czeisler CA, Duffy JF, Shanahan TL, et al. Stability, precision, and near-24-hour period of the human circadian pacemaker. Science 1999;284(5423):2177–81.
2. Eliott AL, Mills JN, Waterhouse JM. A man with too long a day. J Physiol 1971; 212(2):30P–1P.
3. Flynn-Evans EE, Tabandeh H, Skene DJ, et al. Circadian rhythm disorders and melatonin production in 127 blind women with and without light perception. J Biol Rhythms 2014;29(3):215–24.
4. Hayakawa T, Uchiyama M, Kamei Y, et al. Clinical analyses of sighted patients with non-24-hour sleep-wake syndrome: a study of 57 consecutively diagnosed cases. Sleep 2005;28(8):945–52.
5. Malkani RG, Abbott SM, Reid KJ, et al. Diagnostic and treatment challenges of sighted non-24-hour sleep-wake disorder. J Clin Sleep Med 2018;14(4): 603–13.
6. Gooley JJ, Lu J, Chou TC, et al. Melanopsin in cells of origin of the retinohypothalamic tract. Nat Neurosci 2001;4(12):1165.
7. Lockley SW, Skene DJ, Arendt J, et al. Relationship between melatonin rhythms and visual loss in the blind. J Clin Endocrinol Metab 1997;82(11):3763–70.

8. Emens JS, Lewy AJ, Lefler BJ, et al. Relative coordination to unknown "weak zeitgebers" in free-running blind individuals. J Biol Rhythms 2005;20(2): 159–67.

9. Kitamura S, Hida A, Enomoto M, et al. Intrinsic circadian period of sighted patients with circadian rhythm sleep disorder, free-running type. Biol Psychiatry 2013;73(1):63–9.

10. Hida A, Ohsawa Y, Kitamura S, et al. Evaluation of circadian phenotypes utilizing fibroblasts from patients with circadian rhythm sleep disorders. Transl Psychiatry 2017;7(4):e1106.

11. Uchiyama M, Okawa M, Shibui K, et al. Altered phase relation between sleep timing and core body temperature rhythm in delayed sleep phase syndrome and non-24-hour sleep-wake syndrome in humans. Neurosci Lett 2000;294(2): 101–4.

12. Nakamura K, Hashimoto S, Honma S, et al. A sighted man with non-24-hour sleep-wake syndrome shows damped plasma melatonin rhythm. Psychiatry Clin Neurosci 1997;51(3):115–9.

13. Sateia M. The international classification of sleep disorders: diagnostic and coding manual. 2nd edition. Darien (IL): American Academy of Sleep Medicine; 2014.

14. Folkard S, Arendt J, Aldhous M, et al. Melatonin stabilises sleep onset time in a blind man without entrainment of cortisol or temperature rhythms. Neurosci Lett 1990;113(2):193–8.

15. Sack RL, Lewy AJ, Blood ML, et al. Melatonin administration to blind people: phase advances and entrainment. J Biol Rhythms 1991;6(3):249–61.

16. Lockley SW, Skene DJ, James K, et al. Melatonin administration can entrain the free-running circadian system of blind subjects. J Endocrinol 2000;164(1):R1–6.

17. Lewy AJ, Hasler BP, Emens JS, et al. Pretreatment circadian period in free-running blind people may predict the phase angle of entrainment to melatonin. Neurosci Lett 2001;313(3):158–60.

18. Sack RL, Brandes RW, Kendall AR, et al. Entrainment of free-running circadian rhythms by melatonin in blind people. N Engl J Med 2000;343(15):1070–7.

19. Lewy AJ, Bauer VK, Hasler BP, et al. Capturing the circadian rhythms of free-running blind people with 0.5 mg melatonin. Brain Res 2001;918(1–2):96–100.

20. Hack LM, Lockley SW, Arendt J, et al. The effects of low-dose 0.5-mg melatonin on the free-running circadian rhythms of blind subjects. J Biol Rhythms 2003; 18(5):420–9.

21. Lewy AJ, Emens JS, Sack RL, et al. Low, but not high, doses of melatonin entrained a free-running blind person with a long circadian period. Chronobiol Int 2002;19(3):649–58.

22. Lockley SW, Dressman MA, Licamele L, et al. Tasimelteon for non-24-hour sleep-wake disorder in totally blind people (SET and RESET): two multicentre, randomised, double-masked, placebo-controlled phase 3 trials. Lancet 2015; 386(10005):1754–64.

23. Nakamura K, Hashimoto S, Honma S, et al. Daily melatonin intake resets circadian rhythms of a sighted man with non-24-hour sleep-wake syndrome who lacks the nocturnal melatonin rise. Psychiatry Clin Neurosci 1997;51(3):121–7.

24. Hoban TM, Sack RL, Lewy AJ, et al. Entrainment of a free-running human with bright light? Chronobiol Int 1989;6(4):347–53.

25. Oren DA, Giesen HA, Wehr TA. Restoration of detectable melatonin after entrainment to a 24-hour schedule in a 'free-running' man. Psychoneuroendocrinology 1997;22(1):39–52.

26. Watanabe T, Kajimura N, Kato M, et al. Case of a non-24 h sleep-wake syndrome patient improved by phototherapy. Psychiatry Clin Neurosci 2000; 54(3):369–70.
27. Hayakawa T, Kamei Y, Urata J, et al. Trials of bright light exposure and melatonin administration in a patient with non-24 hour sleep-wake syndrome. Psychiatry Clin Neurosci 1998;52(2):261–2.

Irregular Sleep-Wake Rhythm Disorder

Temitayo Oyegbile, MD, PhD[a],*, Aleksandar Videnovic, MD, MSc[b]

KEYWORDS

- Sleep • Circadian • Irregular sleep-wake • Melatonin • Light therapy

KEY POINTS

- Irregular sleep-wake rhythm disorder is characterized by lack of clear major sleep-wake pattern.
- The disorder affects children and adults and is common in individuals with neurodevelopmental delay and neurodegenerative and psychiatric disorders.
- Actigraphy and sleep diaries are used in establishing a diagnosis.
- Treatment modalities encompass use of melatonin, supplemental light exposure, and behavioral modifications aimed at consolidation of sleep-wake rhythm.

IRREGULAR SLEEP-WAKE RHYTHM DISORDER

Patients with irregular sleep-wake rhythm disorder (ISWRD) report difficulties synchronizing their sleep time with that of societal norms.[1] The absence of clear circadian rhythm of sleep-wake leads to irregular periods of sleep during both day and night.[1] As such, patients with this disorder experience notable daytime sleepiness at random times of the day, not associated with a physiologic homeostatic or circadian rhythm pattern. A patient has irregular fragmented sleep over the 24-hour cycle, with the longest sleep periods less than 4 hours each.[2] The longest sleep times usually are from 2:00 AM to 6:00 AM. Total sleep time usually is within the normal range for age within a 24-hour period; however, these patients are unable to consolidate their daily sleep into a single 6-hour to 8-hour period.[1] As a result, this disorder is characterized by a lack of a clearly defined circadian sleep and wake cycle. These patients frequently are in conflict with societal norms and daytime activities. This frequently results in overall sleep restriction because there is an inability to attain adequate sleep of 6 hours to 8 hours during usual nighttime/sleep hours.[3]

Disclosure Statement: Dr. Videnovic discloses support from the grant 5R01NS099055 from the NIH/NINDS.

[a] Georgetown University, MedStar St. Mary's Sleep Lab, Georgetown University Medical Center, 3800 Reservoir Road, Washington, DC 20007, USA; [b] MGH Neurological Clinical Research Institute, 165 Cambridge Street, Suite 600, Boston, MA 02114, USA
* Corresponding author.
E-mail address: too3@georgetown.edu

PREVALENCE

The prevalence of this disorder is unknown but it is estimated to be rare.[1] There are no known gender differences; however, the disorder is prevalent in the elderly, especially among those affected by neurodegenerative disorders. It also commonly found is in children with developmental delay.

PATHOGENESIS

The exact pathogenesis of ISWRD is not fully understood; however, it is believed that a dysfunction within the central processes involved in generation and maintenance of circadian rhythms is responsible.[3] Depending on the disorder type, the development of irregular sleep-wake patterns may be due to changes within the suprachiasmatic nucleus (SCN) or changes to the input that is received by the SCN. A reduction in exposure to zeitgebers, such as light and/or impaired transmission of light signaling to the SCN, as well as changes in melatonin secretion may be culprits of ISWRD. Low daytime light exposure has been associated with increased wake times at night.[4,5] Alterations in social environment also may be responsible for ISWRD. Irregular social schedules, decreased mobility, and adverse effects of medications on sleep as well as increased daytime napping all may play a role. Genetic factors have been implicated in disorders associated with ISWRD, including neurodegenerative disorders, such as Alzheimer disease (AD).[2]

SYMPTOMS

Individuals with ISWRD complain of insomnia or excessive sleepiness associated with multiple (3 or more) irregularly scheduled naps throughout the day, each of varying duration. The insomnia frequently is a sleep maintenance–type insomnia.[3] This can be one of the more onerous disorders for caregivers to deal with. In addition, individuals with this disorder complain of inability to participate in usual daytime activities for prolonged periods of time due to their excessive daytime sleepiness.[2]

DIAGNOSIS

Actigraphy along with a sleep diary over a 7-day to 14-day period is the most useful diagnostic option currently.[1] An actigraph shows a disturbed low-amplitude circadian rhythm with a loss of a normal diurnal sleep-wake patterns (**Fig. 1**). The actigraph also shows at least 3 distinct sleep periods over a 24-hour period. It is imperative that this disorder be distinguished from other sleep disorders associated with poor sleep hygiene and voluntary maintenance of an irregular sleep schedule, such as shift work or jet lag.[1]

TREATMENT

Measures aimed at consolidation of the sleep-cycle are at the core of interventions for ISWRD. The goal is to enhance the amplitude of circadian rhythms and align them to the external physical environment.[1] Treatment involves timed supplemental light exposure, melatonin, and behavioral interventions (**Table 1**). Mixed modality approaches can be used and emphasize use of simultaneous interventions that may produce more robust circadian amplitude and consolidation of sleep-wake cycles. Strategies may include increasing exposure to bright light and staying

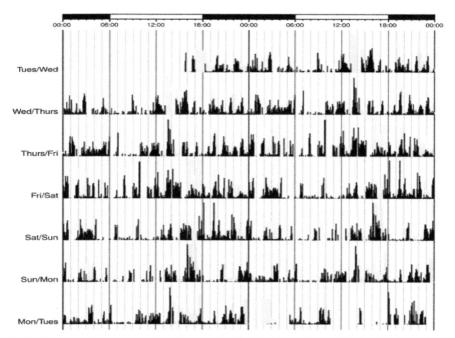

Fig. 1. Typical actigraph seen in patients with ISWRD. (*From* Malkani R, Zee PC. Basic circadian rhythms and circadian sleep disorders. In: Atlas of Sleep Medicine, 2014, 2nd edition; with permission.)

out of the bed during the day, enforcing strict bedtime routines, eliminating noise, and reducing lighting in the bedroom overnight. In children and adults with psychomotor developmental delay, melatonin in doses of 2-mg to 20-mg may improve and consolidate sleep patterns as well as reduce sleep during daytime. Similarly, melatonin, 2 mg, administered at bedtime resulted in improved sleep in individuals with schizophrenia. Melatonin should be avoided in elderly patients with dementia.[2] These individuals may benefit from structured daily activities, bright light exposure, and increased daytime social interactions to improve alertness during the day. Overall, sedatives are not recommended for the treatment of ISWRD. Exercise may be helpful during the daytime; however, exercise alone may not sufficiently treat the disorder. Recent evidence suggests that increasing exposure to a cognitively enriched environment during the daytime may improve symptoms significantly.[3] Studies also suggest that a combination of bright light therapy, chronotherapy, and vitamin B_{12} may be beneficial.[1] Light exposure of 3000 lux to 5000 lux for 2 hours every morning over 4 weeks can improve daytime alertness but may not be as effective in consolidating nighttime sleep. This light exposure may also reduce sundowning behavior in AD patients.[3]

PRACTICE GUIDELINES FROM THE AMERICAN ACADEMY OF SLEEP MEDICINE

There is a clear need for the development of novel treatment modalities, and there is ongoing research to address these concerns.[3] Based on the current limited evidence

Table 1
Current treatment recommendations for irregular sleep-wake rhythm disorder

Population	Treatment	Results/Outcomes
Elderly with and without dementia	Light	Daytime light exposure (2500 lux) may increase total sleep time at night.[6]
	Melatonin	Randomized controlled trials have shown no improvement in sleep and may worsen mood.[7,8]
	Mixed-modality treatment	Morning bright light (>10,000 lux), low-level physical activity, structured bedtime routine, and reduction of light and noise at night can improve sleep.[5,9]
Children	Light	Morning bright light (4500 lux) normalized the sleep-wake cycle.[10]
	Melatonin	Doses ranging from 1 mg to 5 mg have improved sleep-wake patterns.[11]
	Mixed-modality treatment	Environmental modification, positive bedtime routines, calming activities, and stimulus control are recommended.[12,13]
Psychiatric Disorders	Light	Daytime bright light exposure (up to 10,000 lux) improved sleep-wake cycle.[14]
	Melatonin	Melatonin, 2 mg, at bedtime improved sleep.[15]

available in the literature, however, the American Academy of Sleep Medicine (AASM) has recommended the following practice guidelines:

1. Clinicians should treat ISWRD in elderly patients with dementia with light therapy. (WEAK EVIDENCE)
2. Clinicians should avoid the use of sedating or sleep-promoting medications to treat elderly patients with dementia and ISWRD. (STRONG EVIDENCE)
3. Clinicians should avoid the use of melatonin as a treatment of ISWRD in elderly patients with dementia. (WEAK EVIDENCE)
4. Clinicians should use strategically timed orally administered melatonin as a treatment of ISWRD in children and adolescents with neurologic disorders. (WEAK EVIDENCE)
5. Clinicians should avoid the use of combined treatments consisting of light therapy in combination with melatonin in elderly ISWRD patients with dementia. (WEAK EVIDENCE)
6. There are no specific recommendations from AASM for the use of the following treatment options to manage ISWRD:
   a. Prescribed sleep-wake scheduling
   b. Timed physical activity/exercise
   c. Strategic avoidance of light
   d. Wakefulness-promoting medications
   e. Other somatic interventions

IRREGULAR SLEEP-WAKE DISORDER IN SPECIAL POPULATIONS

ISWRD frequently is observed in neurodegenerative disorders and brain injury.[2] It also is associated with children with psychomotor developmental delay and autistic spectrum disorders. In these disorders, irregular sleep and wake patterns are believed associated with dysfunction in the central processes associated with the maintenance of circadian rhythms.[3] Angelman syndrome and Smith-Magenis syndrome are examples of child neurodevelopmental disorders characterized by irregular sleep pattern and inversion of the sleep-wake cycles that may go along with decreased amplitude of melatonin rhythm. Neurodegenerative disorders, such as dementias, are associated with ISWRD. Elderly individuals with AD may experience severe sleep fragmentation with low circadian rhythm amplitude, especially if they have symptoms of sundowning. Elderly individuals in nursing homes also may experience similar disorders, which may be due to a lack of regular exposure to bright light and social schedules.[2]

Older Adults With and Without Dementia

Up to 70% of older adults complain of sleep disturbances from irregular sleep-wake cycles.[16] The prevalence of irregular sleep-wake cycle is even higher in a population of AD and related dementias. These individuals have diminished amplitude of the rest-activity rhythm, with poorly consolidated sleep and frequently inverted sleep-wake cycles. Evidence suggests a reduction in neuronal activation of the SCN in older adults. Melatonin rhythm becomes less robust in AD. These changes lead to an alteration of circadian rhythm patterns and regularity. Ultimately, the SCN becomes less responsive to light leading to less entrainment of the sleep-wake cycle.[17] This circadian misalignment can have significant consequences on sleep.

Assisted living facilities tend to provide limited bright light exposure to their residents; middle-aged adults experience approximately 60 minutes of bright light exposure during the day whereas older adults especially with dementia and/or in nursing homes can be exposed to less than 2 minutes of bright light daily.[18] Even among older adults who deny suffering any sleep disturbance, it is clear that irregular disrupted sleep-wake cycles can significantly impair cognitive function.[19] Assisted living facilities would benefit from bright lighting to improve irregular sleep-wake rhythms in the elderly. Riemersma-van der Lek and colleagues[7] evaluated assisted living facilities that were randomly assigned to emit bright white light (1000 lux) or dim light (300 lux) in their ceiling fixtures within the common areas during the daytime. Individuals in brightly lit facilities had lower total sleep time, reduced cognitive deficits, and improved depression symptoms at 6 weeks and 6 months. In this population, non-pharmacologic interventions to improve the sleep-wake cycle was key to improving quality of life.[5] Specifically, bright light exposure (especially sunlight) increased physical activity and structured bedtime routines, and elimination of nighttime noise and light played crucial roles in improving irregular sleep-wake cycles. Bright light exposure to treat ISWRD is most effective in individuals with relatively good vision.[20] There seems to be little role for pharmacologic interventions in this population. A meta-analysis assessing the benefits and risks of sedative/hypnotic interventions in this population with irregular sleep-wake cycles showed that the benefits do not clearly outweigh the significantly increased risk associated with the constant use of these medications.[21] There may be a role for melatonin, however, in treating the ISWRD. Riemersma-van der Lek and colleagues[7] found that a combination of bright light exposure and melatonin treatment led to improved sleep efficiency, reduced nighttime activity, and improved cognitive and behavioral function.[7] The AASM, however, currently does not recommend combination therapy.[3]

In addition to improving sleep, both cognition and behavior are improved when light exposure is optimized among older adults with dementia. Light exposure, especially in the evening, can decrease nighttime activity significantly, including eloping/walking. In addition, agitated behaviors and sundowning were significantly improved with 1 hour of bright light (10,000 lux) every morning for 2 weeks.[22,23] These findings are not unique to AD. Studies looking at other dementia types, including vascular dementia, showed similar findings.[24] The time of day of light exposure seems to have a significant effect as well. Morning light leads to improved sleep better than evening light exposure and all-day light exposure.[25] In general, there are minimal gender differences; however, evidence suggests that older women have a better improvement in depressive symptoms with morning light exposure compared with older men.[25]

Overall, it is clear that supplemental light exposure as an intervention to treat ISWRD in the elderly with and without dementia can be beneficial. In addition, strategic light exposure in long-term care/assisted living facilities is important to improve sleep, depression, behavior, and cognition in older adults with dementias.[26]

Parkinson Disease

Parkinson disease (PD) is a movement disorder characterized by tremors, slowness, and stiffness. In addition to these motor manifestations of the disease, several nonmotor manifestations of PD negatively affect quality of life and safety of PD patients. Among these nonmotor manifestations, impaired sleep and alertness are common. Excessive sleepiness affects up to 30% of patients with PD.[27] Sleep fragmentation is the most common sleep disturbance in PD. These impairments of alertness and sleep continuity are the bases for irregular sleep-wake rhythms in PD. The etiology of poor sleep and poor alertness in PD is multifactorial and encompasses overnight emergence of motor symptoms, effects of dopaminergic medications, coexistent primary sleep, and psychiatric disorders as well as effects of the primary neurodegenerative process underlying PD. Circadian dysfunction has emerged as a novel factor underlying irregular sleep-wake rhythms in individuals with PD. Circadian melatonin rhythm, which is an accepted marker of the endogenous circadian system, is dampened in individuals with PD.[28] This observation is suggestive of low circadian amplitude and has provided an opportunity for development of circadian-based interventions that target impaired sleep-wake cycles in PD. In this regard, several studies have documented beneficial effects of light therapy on sleep quality and sleepiness in PD.[29–31]

Psychiatric Disorders

Individuals with psychiatric disorders, such as bipolar disorder and schizophrenia, frequently report sleep disturbances. Poor control of and more exacerbations of these disorders are associated with irregular sleep-wake rhythm. Irregular sleep is one of the most important signs of the emergence of a hypomanic/manic episode[32] and schizophrenia exacerbations.[33,34] A recent review showed that individuals that are high risk for bipolar disorder report persistent irregularity in their sleep-wake rhythms.[35] As a result, irregular sleep patterns could be used as a marker to identify changes in disease patterns, leading to exacerbations.[32] Further research is necessary to fully characterize this relationship and to determine the best intervention options for this population.

Irregular Young Adult Sleepers

ISWRD also has the substantial consequences on the general population regardless of age or mental health disorders. Irregular sleep-wake patterns in a young relatively healthy undergraduate population can have significant effects on academic performance.[36] Young individuals with adequate sleep duration but irregular sleep patterns show poorer performance in real-world social and academic settings compared with regular sleepers. In addition, individuals with irregular sleep tend to have delayed sleep timing and more daytime naps, which can perpetuate the irregularity of sleep-wake patterns. The irregular sleep also can have effects on sleep physiology because there is evidence of delayed onset of melatonin secretion despite appropriate circadian and homeostatic cues.[36]

Autism

Children with autism tend to have irregular sleep-wake patterns, including early awakening in the morning and later sleep times in the evening.[37] These children tend to have significant variability in total daily sleep time with large day-to-day variations. These sleep concerns tend to be worse in children younger than 4 years of age. Nighttime awakening with significant nighttime activity frequently is reported. Children with autism also frequently take daytime naps, regardless of age. This variability in sleep leads to irregular sleep-wake patterns and fragmented sleep duration.[37] These children are much less likely to show signs of delayed sleep-phase syndrome or advanced sleep-phase syndrome. As a result, a clear characterization of sleep patterns in children with autism has yet to be defined. Children with autism seem to have a bifurcation of the sleep-wake cycle with increased sensitivity to external noise and irregular sleep onset and offset.[37] This may be due to an altered balance of the circadian and homeostatic signals associated with sleep. Overall, children with autism tend to have shorter sleep periods over a 24-hour period compared with typically developing children.[38,39]

Animal studies show that the disturbance in circadian rhythm in autism may be related to dysfunction in the serotonergic system in the brain.[39,40] There is a reduced serotonin transporter binding capacity in children with autism; this may be the result of a primary deficit in melatonin synthesis, leading to accumulation of upstream serotonin. As a result, exogenous melatonin administration may be beneficial and therapeutic. With older age, the irregular sleep pattern begins to improve but tends to remain a significant trait of the disorder throughout the life span.

SUMMARY

In conclusion, ISWRD is considered a rare disorder, which is concentrated in specific populations with comorbid neurologic/psychiatric disorders. This disorder most commonly is noted in elderly patients with dementias but also is commonly observed in young children with notable neurologic disorders, such as autism spectrum disorder. Researchers have suggested that ISWRD likely is a manifestation of dysfunction of the sleep-wake–generating mechanisms within the brain. Because of the rarity of this disorder as well as the heterogeneity of comorbid neurologic conditions among individuals with ISWRD, a clear characterization and understanding of the underlying mechanisms have eluded researchers to this point. As a consequence, the treatments options available currently remain limited. Currently, the best options for treatment of this disorder are light therapy among the elderly and melatonin therapy in younger individuals with neurologic disorders. The focus of ISWRD research currently is to find novel treatment interventions that can improve daytime function and cognition in individuals with this disorder.

REFERENCES

1. Abbott SM, Zee PC. Irregular sleep-wake rhythm disorder. Sleep Med Clin 2015; 10:517–22.
2. Pavlova M. Circadian rhythm sleep-wake disorders. Continuum 2017;23: 1051–63.
3. Auger RR, Burgess HJ, Emens JS, et al. Clinical practice guideline for the treatment of intrinsic circadian rhythm sleep-wake disorders: advanced sleep-wake phase disorder (ASWPD), delayed sleep-wake phase disorder (DSWPD), non-24-hour sleep-wake rhythm disorder (N24SWD), and irregular sleep-wake

disorder (ISWRD). An update for 2015: An American Academy of Sleep Medicine clinical practice guideline. J Clin Sleep Med 2015;11:1199–236.

4. Figueiro MG. Light, sleep and circadian rhythms in older adults with Alzheimer's disease and related dementias. Neurodegener Dis Manag 2017;7:119–45.

5. Alessi CA, Martin JL, Webber AP, et al. Randomized, controlled trial of a nonpharmacological intervention to improve abnormal sleep/wake patterns in nursing home residents. J Am Geriatr Soc 2005;53:803–10.

6. Ancoli-Israel S, Gehrman P, Martin JL, et al. Increased light exposure consolidates sleep and strengthens circadian rhythms in severe Alzheimer's disease patients. Behav Sleep Med 2003;1:22–36.

7. Riemersma-van der Lek RF, Swaab DF, Twisk J, et al. Effect of bright light and melatonin on cognitive and noncognitve function in elderly residents of group care facilities: a randomized controlled trial. JAMA 2008;299:2642–55.

8. Serfaty M, Kennell-Webb S, Warner J, et al. Double blind randomized placebo controlled trial of low melatonin for sleep disorders in dementia. Int J Geriatr Psychiatry 2002;17:1120–7.

9. McCurry SM, Gibbons LE, Logsdon RG, et al. Nighttime insomnia treatment and education for Alzheimer's disease: a randomized, controlled trial. J Am Geriatr Soc 2005;53:793–802.

10. Guilleminault C, McCann CC, Quera-Salva M, et al. Light therapy as treatment of dyschronosis in brain impaired children. Eur J Pediatr 1993;152:754–9.

11. Esposito S, Laino D, D'Alonzo R, et al. Pediatric sleep disturbances and treatment with melatonin. J Transl Med 2019;17:77.

12. Souders MC, Zavodny S, Eriksen W, et al. Sleep in children with autism spectrum disorder. Curr Psychiatry Rep 2017;19:34.

13. Cuomo BM, Vaz S, Lee EAL, et al. Effectiveness of sleep-based interventions for children with autism spectrum disorder: a meta-synthesis. Pharmacotherapy 2017;37:555–78.

14. Sheaves B, Freeman D, Isham L, et al. Stabilising sleep for patients admitted at acute crisis to a psychiatric hospital (OWLS): an assessor-blind pilot randomized controlled trial. Psychol Med 2018;48:1694–704.

15. Shamir E, Laudon M, Barak Y, et al. Melatonin improves sleep quality of patients with chronic schizophrenia. J Clin Psychiatry 2000;61:373–7.

16. Van Someren EJ. Circadian and sleep disturbances in the elderly. Exp Gerontol 2000;35:1229–37.

17. Swaab DF, Dubelaar EJ, Hofman MA, et al. Brain aging and Alzheimer's disease; use it or lose it. Prog Brain Res 2002;138:343–73.

18. Ancoli-Israel S, Kripke DF. Now I lay me down to sleep: the problem with sleep fragmentation in elderly and demented residents of nursing homes. Bull Clin Neurosci 1989;54:127–32.

19. Moe KE, Vitiello MV, Larsen LH, et al. Symposium: cognitive processes and sleep disturbances: sleep/wake patterns in Alzheimer's disease: relationships with cognition and function. J Sleep Res 1995;4:15–20.

20. Agorastos A, Skevas C, Matthaei M, et al. Depression, anxiety, and disturbed sleep in glaucoma. J Neuropsychiatry Clin Neurosci 2013;25:205–13.

21. Glass J, Lanctot KL, Herrmann N, et al. Sedative hyponotics in older people with insomnia: meta-analysis of risks and benefits. BMJ 2005;331:1169.

22. Satlin A, Volicer L, Ross V, et al. Bright light treatment for behavioral and sleep distubances in patients with Alzheimer's disease. Am J Psychiatry 1992;149: 1028–32.

23. Lyketosos CG, Lindell Veiel L, Baker A, et al. A randomized, controlled trial of bright light therapy for agitated behaviors in dementia patients residing in long-term care. Int J Geriatr Psychiatry 1999;14:520–5.

24. Mishima K, Hishikawa Y, Okawa M. Randomized, dim light controlled, crossover test of morning bright light therapy for rest-activity rhythm disorders in patients with vascular dementia and dementia of Alzheimer's type. Chronobiol Int 1998; 15:647–54.

25. Hickman SE, Barrick AL, Williams CS, et al. The effect of ambient bright light therapy on depressive symptoms in persons with dementia. J Am Geriatr Soc 2007; 55:1817–24.

26. Figueiro MG, Plitnick B, Lok A, et al. Tailored lighting intervention improves measures of sleep, depression, and agitation in persons with Alzheimer's disease and related dementia living in long-term care facilities. Clin Interv Aging 2014;9: 1527–37.

27. Chahine L, Amara A, Videnovic A. A systematic review of the literature on disorders of sleep and wakefulness in Parkinson's disease from 2005-2015. Sleep Med Rev 2016. https://doi.org/10.1016/j.smrv.2016.08.001.

28. Videnovic A, Noble C, Reid K, et al. Circadian melatonin rhythm and excessive daytime sleepiness in Parkinson's disease. JAMA Neurol 2014;71(4):463–9.

29. Videnovic A, Klerman EB, Wang W, et al. Timed light therapy for sleep and daytime sleepiness associated with parkinson disease: a randomized clinical trial. JAMA Neurol 2017;74(4):411–8.

30. Willis GL, Turner EJ. Primary and secondary features of Parkinson's disease improve with strategic exposure to bright light: a case series study. Chronobiology Int 2007;24(3):521–37.

31. Paus S, Schmitz-Hubsch T, Wullner U, et al. Bright light therapy in Parkinson's disease: a pilot study. Mov Disord 2007;22(10):1495–8.

32. Kanady JC, Soehnera AM, Harvey AG. A retrospective examination of sleep disturbance across the course of bipolar disorder. J Sleep Disord Ther 2015;4: 1000193.

33. Chung KF, Poon YPY, Ng TK, et al. Correlates of sleep irregularity in schizophrenia. Psychiatry Res 2018;270:705–14.

34. Fukuda T, Haraguchi A, Takahashi M, et al. A randomized, double-blind and placebo-controlled crossover trial on the effect of l-ornithine ingestion on the human circadian clock. Chronobiol Int 2018;3:1–11.

35. Melo MC, Garcia RF, Linhares Neto VB, et al. Sleep and circadian alterations in people at risk for bipolar disorder: a systematic review. J Psychiatr Res 2016; 83:211–9.

36. Phillips AJK, Clerx WM, O'Brien CS, et al. Irregular sleep/wake patterns are associated with poorer academic performance and delayed circadian and sleep/wake timing. Sci Rep 2017;7:3216.

37. Matsuura H, Tateno K, Aou S. Dynamical properties of the two-process model for sleep-wake cycles in infantile autism. Cogn Neurodyn 2008;2:221–8.

38. Goodlin-Jones BL, Tang K, Liu J, et al. Sleep patterns in preschool children with autism, developmental delay, and typical development. J Am Acad Child Adolesc Psychiatry 2008;47:932–40.

39. Tsujino N, Nakatani Y, Seki Y, et al. Abnormality of circadian rhythm accompanied by an increase in frontal cortex serotonin in animal model of autism. Neurosci Res 2007;57:289–95.

40. Cortesi F, Giannotti F, Ivanenko A, et al. Sleep in children with autistic spectrum disorder. Sleep Med 2010;11:659–64.

Shift Work Disorder

Philip Cheng, PhD*,1, Christopher Drake, PhD1

KEYWORDS

- Shift work • Circadian rhythms • Sleep • Sleepiness

KEY POINTS

- Shift work disorder (SWD) is common among shift workers.
- SWD has adverse consequences for health and psychological functioning.
- Assessments for SWD have been improving with technological and scientific advances.
- Clinical management for SWD should rely on both pharmacologic and nonpharmacologic approaches.

INTRODUCTION

In a globalizing economy with demands for 24-hour consumer service, the impact of shift work is increasingly relevant. Shift work may encompass work schedules deviating from the traditional day shift (typically starting between 7 AM and 10 AM), and is generally categorized as fixed night, early morning, late afternoon/evening, or rotating shifts. Estimates suggest that between 15% and 30% of the European and American workforce is engaged in shift work,[1,2] with some indication that the prevalence of shift work is increasing. For example, comparison of shift work from 2000 to 2014 showed consistent increases (4%–13% increase) in individuals reporting working a morning, evening, or night shift.[3]

Shifts that deviate significantly from the traditional work schedule inevitably require employees to work at times when sleep typically occurs (ie, during the night), and sleep during the daytime. Many shift workers have trouble adapting to this scheduling, leading to poor or insufficient daytime sleep and excessive nocturnal sleepiness during their work shifts. In fact, approximately 10% of the US workforce (~3 million workers) experience sleep disturbance and sleepiness severe enough to meet criteria for shift work disorder (SWD[4]). As determined by the International Classification of Sleep Disorders, third edition[5] (ICSD-3), SWD is characterized by insomnia and/or excessive sleepiness during wakefulness, typically accompanied by a reduction of total sleep time.

Disclosure Statement: Dr. Cheng received funding from the National Heart Lung and Blood Institute (K23HL138166). Dr. Drake received funding from the National Institute of Mental Health (R56MH115150) and the National Institute of Nursing Research (R01NR013959).
Sleep Disorders and Research Center, Henry Ford Health System, Detroit, MI 48202, USA
1 Present address: 39450 West 12 Mile Road, Novi, MI 48377.
* Corresponding author.
E-mail address: pcheng1@hfhs.org

Neurol Clin 37 (2019) 563–577
https://doi.org/10.1016/j.ncl.2019.03.003
0733-8619/19/© 2019 Elsevier Inc. All rights reserved.
neurologic.theclinics.com

THE BIOLOGY OF SHIFT WORK DISORDER

Although many shift workers experience difficulties in work performance and health complications, not everyone reports such difficulties. The prevailing theory is that individuals experience difficulties with the shift work schedule due to disruptions to one or both independent biological processes that regulate sleep and sleepiness. The first is a *misalignment* between their internal circadian rhythms and their work and sleep schedules. Specifically, the human sleep/wake system is partially governed by an internal biological clock that regulates a host of physiologic and psychological functions (including alertness and sleep propensity) that fluctuate across the 24-hour day. This internal clock is synchronized to the 24-hour day by an individual's exposure to natural sunlight (or other source of bright light), and cycles relatively independent of direct effects from sleep. When workers attempt to sleep and work out of phase with the rhythms of their internal biological clock, they commonly experience acutely disrupted daytime sleep and excessive nocturnal sleepiness that may lead to chronic difficulties with sleep and wakefulness.

In addition to circadian rhythms, sleep and wakefulness are also governed by a sleep-wake–dependent process. This process is characterized as sleep pressure that builds with wakefulness and dissipates with sleep. As such, sleepiness also may occur as a result of an excessive buildup of sleep pressure from prolonged wakefulness or inadequate dissipation of sleep pressure due to curtailed sleep. Because shift workers often experience sleep disruption and may also reduce their opportunity for sleep when sleeping during the day, they are also prone to excessive sleepiness due to a heightened sleep pressure.

CONSEQUENCES OF SHIFT WORK
Health

Because most physiologic systems have a circadian component and are also impacted by sleep, shift workers often experience a cascade of consequences beyond sleep disruption and sleepiness. This includes increased risk for medical morbidities due to dysregulated functioning of a range of physiologic systems. For example, hunger, food preference, and metabolism are important biological processes that have a strong circadian component. Consequently, shift work has been posited to increase unhealthy eating, such as increased consumption of calorically dense foods. An epidemiologic study found that workers on a rotating shift show increased odds (odds ratio 1.57; 95% confidence interval [CI] 1.12–2.21) of obesity, with a significant trend of increased odds with longer duration of shift work.[6] However, a meta-analysis of studies comparing shift workers and day workers did not find significant differences in energy intake,[7] suggesting that obesity in shift work may be related to meal timing and circadian variations in energy metabolism.

One consequence of mistimed eating may be impaired metabolic functioning, such as reduced glucose tolerance. One laboratory study found that acute circadian misalignment of sleep and food intake in healthy adults was associated with an exaggerated postprandial glucose response, with some participants showing values consistent with a prediabetic or diabetic state.[8] Furthermore, a systematic review found consistent evidence for a moderate increase in risk for diabetes among shift workers.[9] The largest study of almost 200,000 night-shift nurses showed that the hazard ratio for diabetes was 1.06 (95% CI 1.01–1.11) for those with 3 to 9 years of night-shift exposure, and 1.24 (95% CI 1.13–1.37) for more than 20 years of night-shift exposure,[10] suggesting that physiologic abnormalities may result in medical morbidities through a process that may take years or even decades to develop.

Shift work has also been implicated in risk for the development of specific forms of cancer. The International Agency for Research on Cancer declared shift work that involved circadian disruption to be a "probable" carcinogen in 2007 based on basic science using animal models. Although epidemiologic studies have not shown consistent evidence in humans, a recent meta-analysis of 61 studies found a positive association between shift work and cancer.[11] Indeed, results suggested that every 5 years of night-shift work was associated with a 3.3% increase in the risk of breast cancer in women. Other large prospective studies have noted an overall 36% to 60% increased risk for breast cancer. Although studies of the underlying mechanisms are still under way, it has been suggested that a mediating factor in the relationship between shift work and cancer risk may be a reduction of free radical scavenging related to melatonin suppression from exposure to nocturnal light. In turn, the reduction of free radical scavenging leads to a reduced tumor-inhibition.[12,13]

Psychological Functioning in Shift Work

The compounding effects of sleep deprivation and circadian misalignment also leaves many shift workers vulnerable to deficits in the cognitive domain, which greatly impact occupational performance and have consequences for productivity and employee safety, as well as public safety. Despite its importance, research delineating the *specific* cognitive vulnerabilities associated with shift work is still nascent. Extant research has focused on vigilance as measured by the psychomotor vigilance task, with many studies showing increased attentional lapses and slowed reaction time during the biological night.[14–16]

Emerging evidence also suggests that specific cognitive components may be differentially associated with psychophysiology versus symptom presentation.[17] In a study that dismantled cognitive flexibility into the subcomponents of attending to new stimuli versus suppression of old stimuli, results showed that attentional flexibility for new stimuli was most strongly associated with circadian phase as opposed to symptoms of sleepiness or insomnia. Furthermore, symptoms of insomnia versus sleepiness were also differentially associated with specific deficits: whereas shift workers with insomnia symptoms exhibited difficulties in suppressing previous information that is now irrelevant to the task at hand, sleepy shift workers exhibited difficulties repeating previously completed tasks. This finding is consistent with prior research indicating that although shift workers with insomnia show increased cortical activity, they are less attentive to novel stimuli presented in their environment.[18,19] Importantly, the specific components of cognitive flexibility had a differential impact on task performance. Those with difficulties with attentional flexibility for new stimuli took longer to complete tasks, with some requiring 2-times the amount of time for task completion. This has significant implications for efficiency and productivity. In contrast, shift workers exhibiting difficulties with suppression of task-irrelevant stimuli showed reduced accuracy, particularly with greater occurrences of perseverative errors. This also has important implications for productivity and safety. For example, cognitive fixation (ie, inflexibility) was cited as a contributing cause to the 2005 BP America Refinery explosions[20] that killed 15 people and injured another 180. Although this disaster occurred during daytime hours, the refinery relied on shift workers working 12-hour shifts across consecutive days. In addition, investigations tracing events leading up to the explosion also cited errors made during the night shift, and during the transition between shifts as contributing factors.

To date, only 1 study has prospectively examined the effects of *chronic* exposure to shift work on cognitive functioning, and the reversibility of these effects.[21] Overall, the study revealed that exposure to shift work was associated with a 1.6-point decrease in global cognitive performance on a scale of 0 to 100. Assuming a linear decline of cognitive functioning over 30 years for an average 32-year-old, the magnitude of the effect of overall exposure to shift work was equivalent to 4.3 years of age-related decline. However, further analyses comparing exposure duration revealed that exposure to more than 10 years of shift work was associated with greater global declines in cognitive functioning compared with those with 10 or fewer years of exposure to shift work. Specifically, those with more than 10 years of shift work exposure exhibited a 2.5-point decrease (equivalent to 6.5 years of age-related decline) compared with those without exposure to shift work, whereas those with 10 or fewer years of shift work exhibited a 0.9-point decrease (equivalent to 2.4 years of age-related decline). Analyses were also completed to examine how long these cognitive deficits lingered following the transition away from shift work. Findings suggested that those who were within 5 years of exposure to shift work continued to exhibit impairment, whereas those who had more than 5 years of recovery from shift work showed no differences in cognitive functioning compared with those with no history of shift work.

Emotional/Affective Functioning

Given the close relationship among sleep, circadian rhythms, and affective functioning, there has been some concern regarding the deleterious effects that shift work may have on mental/emotional health. Prior research indicates that global affect exhibits a circadian rhythm, with the trough occurring nocturnally, at approximately 0200.[22] This is consistent with evidence that physiologic systems involved in affect and affective regulation (ie, serotonin, norepinephrine, and dopamine) are also under circadian control and exhibit a circadian rhythm (for review, see McClung[23]). Furthermore, there is also evidence that monoaminergic activity (implicated in mood disruption) can be modulated by melatonin activity, which is critical for the functioning of the central circadian pacemaker. This suggests that melatonin activity may have downstream effects for mood and mood regulation, and further indicates that disruptions to the circadian pacemaker may also lead to mood dysregulation.

In line with basic research, qualitative clinical research in night-shift nurses indicates that depression is a common problem in shift workers.[24] Another study also found that nurses on a rotating shift schedule reported moderately greater psychiatric symptoms compared with day-shift nurses (Cohen's d for difference = 0.41).[25] However, a recent systematic review suggests that the accumulating evidence for shift work as a general risk for depression is mixed,[26] with some studies finding increased risk and others do not. One explanation may be that risk for depression in shift work may be more specific to the type of maladjustment to shift work; although common, not all who engage in shift work experience significant impairments in functioning, and those who do may self-select out of occupations with shift work (ie, the "Healthy Worker Effect"). Specifically, a prospective study of individuals transitioning to shift work found that both depression and anxiety 1 year after onset of shift work was mediated by the development of SWD.[27]

Psychosocial Functioning

One important but sometimes neglected domain of the phenomenology of shift work is psychosocial functioning. Indeed, some studies have found that the association between shift work and depression may be accounted for in-part by the psychosocial work conditions,[28–30] particularly for occupations outside of the health sector.[26] A more recent study found that job satisfaction was moderately lower in rotating shift nurses compared with day-shift nurses (Cohen's d for difference = 0.66),[25] whereas another study found that shift workers report feeling less support from managers and leaders.[30] It is also common that employee well-being initiatives offered through the workplace (including social gatherings) are less accessible to shift workers due to scheduling conflicts. On the other hand, there also have been reports that shift workers may develop strong comradery around their uniquely shared challenges.[30,31]

Social engagement also appears to be negatively impacted by shift work. An analysis of time dedicated to social participation in the United Kingdom suggested that shift workers were somewhat less socially engaged.[32] Activities representative of social participation included 8 domains: general engagement with social support networks, helping members of the community (eg, helping neighbor with shopping), civic engagement (eg, attending a town hall), volunteering, attendance at cultural and artistic events, playing sports/games, extracurricular learning, and religious activities. Whereas day workers dedicated an average of 8.25 hours per week toward social participation, shift workers averaged closer to 6.75 hours per week. In addition, a study of time and activities outside of work in a sample of nurses found that 52% of night-shift workers and 27% of evening-shift workers reported rarely or never having spare time,[33] which also likely accounts for the reduced social engagement among shift workers. Given the importance of social connectedness to mental health, it is also likely that mood disturbances associated with shift work are exacerbated by social isolation and reduced social participation.

EVALUATION AND DIAGNOSIS OF SHIFT WORK DISORDER

SWD is defined in the ICSD-3 as follows[5]:

1. There is a report of insomnia and/or excessive sleepiness, accompanied by a reduction of total sleep time, which is associated with a recurring work schedule that overlaps with the usual time for sleep.
2. The symptoms have been present and associated with the shift work schedule for at least 3 months.
3. The symptoms cause clinically significant distress or impairment in mental, physical, social, occupational, education, or other important areas of functioning.
4. Sleep log and actigraphy monitoring (whenever possible and preferably with concurrent measurement of light exposure) for at least 14 days (work and free days) demonstrate a disturbed sleep and wake pattern.
5. The sleep and/or wake disturbance is not better explained by another current sleep disorder, medical or neurologic disorder, mental disorder, medication use, poor sleep hygiene, or substance use disorder.

Essential components for a comprehensive evaluation of SWD would ideally include a clinical interview of sleep history (with assessment of safety risk due to excessive sleepiness) along with use of validated instruments to measure sleep-wake patterns (eg, sleep logs and/or actigraphy). Polysomnography is necessary only if there is a need to rule out other sleep disorders that may be contributing to poor sleep, such as obstructive sleep apnea (OSA).

History

A clinical interview for shift workers should include an assessment of work history, a detailed sleep history, and impairments during wakefulness. A comprehensive work history should include occupation, work schedule (eg, shift start and end times, rotation speed and direction, number of shifts per week, how shifts are assigned/scheduled, how long they have been on the shift system), and the perceived benefits and trade-offs of their shift system.

Sleep patterns should be assessed separately for both on-shift and off-shift periods, as shift workers commonly move their sleep period in accordance with their work schedule. Sleepiness during the night shift also should be assessed, and can be achieved with several instruments. The Insomnia Severity Index (ISI) is commonly used for assessing sleep disturbances and can be applied separately for nighttime versus daytime sleep.[34] A score of ≥10 on the ISI is indicative of clinically significant insomnia. The Epworth Sleepiness Scale is also validated and commonly used for assessing sleepiness during wakefulness, with a score ≥10 indicative of excessive sleepiness.[35]

Use of medications and other substances that directly (eg, hypnotic or wake-promoting agents) or indirectly impact sleep are also important (see **Table 1** for common medications that have sedating/alerting side effects). Performance deficits, including accidental dozing (particularly while driving), are critical to identify.

Table 1
Common medications with sedating and alerting side effects

Common Medications That Have Sedating Side Effects	Common Medications That Have Alerting Side Effects and Can Disrupt Sleep
• First-generation antihistamines (eg, Benadryl) • Sedating antidepressants (eg, mirtazapine, trazodone, amitriptyline) • Anxiolytics (eg, diazepam, lorazepam) • Pain medications (eg, opiates, narcotics) • Sedating anticonvulsants (eg, gabapentin, carbamazepine) • Antipsychotics (eg, quetiapine, risperidone, olanzapine) • Hypnotics (eg, benzodiazepines, nonbenzodiazepine hypnotics, melatonin agonists) • Dopamine agonists for Parkinson disease (eg, pramipexole, ropinirole, pergolide) • Some muscle relaxants (eg, cyclobenzaprine)	• Attention-deficit/hyperactivity disorder medications • Alerting antidepressants (eg, selective serotonin reuptake inhibitors, tricyclic) • Corticosteroids (eg, prednisone, methylprednisolone) • Smoking cessation medications (eg, nicotine patches) • Angiotensin-converting enzyme inhibitors • Diuretics • Ephedrine and pseudoephedrine • Some immunosuppressants (eg, tacrolimus, ciclosporin) • Antineoplastic agents • Thyroid medications (eg, aminophylline)

Consistent with most diagnostic interviews, assessment of SWD also should probe for symptoms of comorbid sleep disorders, such as OSA, narcolepsy, restless legs syndrome/Willis-Ekbom disease, periodic limb movement disorder, and parasomnias. This includes questions about loud or habitual snoring, witnessed pauses in breathing during sleep, cataplexy, hypnagogic hallucinations or sleep paralysis, an uncomfortable urge to move the legs, and abnormal movements or behaviors during sleep.

Sleep Diary

Use of a sleep diary is common in the evaluation of sleep-wake disturbances related to shift work. A sleep diary should be completed prospectively for 2 weeks. Either the 24-hour sleep log or the consensus sleep diary can be used (**Fig. 1** for example of 24-hour sleep log). Although the consensus sleep diary is amenable for calculating common sleep parameters (eg, sleep-onset latency, wake time after sleep onset, sleep efficiency), the 24-hour diary has the advantage of visually depicting the occurrence of sleep bouts in relation to work shifts, as well as change in sleep timing across days. This increases the ease for detection of patterns and thus is more commonly used when circadian rhythm sleep-wake disorders are suspected.

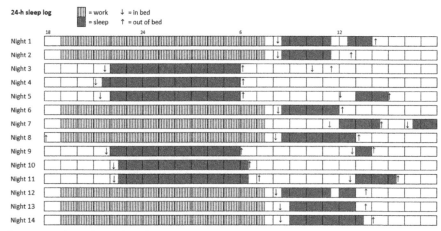

Fig. 1. Sample 24-hour sleep log.

Information from the sleep diary can be used for a detailed characterization of sleep patterns on work days, off days, transition to work days, and transition to off days. Sleep metrics are recorded longitudinally on the sleep diary and can be summarized quantitatively, providing higher resolution compared with retrospective self-report. Quantitative data often include average sleep efficiency, sleep-onset latency, wake timing following sleep onset, frequency of night awakenings, and sleep quality. These variables also can be charted over time to monitor response to treatment.

Actigraphy

Actigraphy is commonly used as a complement to the sleep diary, but may also be a viable alternative to sleep logs in patients who have difficulty with self-reported sleep, or when there are inconsistencies between symptom presentation and self-reported sleep. Actigraphy is usually obtained via a wrist-worn device placed on the nondominant hand, and measures movement and (with some models) light exposure. Actigraphy and has been shown to be comparable to polysomnography for evaluation of total sleep time.[36] Actigraphy also can be a useful outcome measure in evaluating response to treatment for SWD. As with the ISI, attention should be directed to both daytime and nighttime sleep.

Chronotype

History of circadian preference also may be assessed, although this can be complicated by the shift work schedule, especially for those who have worked a nontraditional shift system for extended periods. Circadian preference (otherwise commonly referred to as "chronotype") refers to an underlying tendency for individuals to have a morning preference (eg, "morning lark" or early chronotype) versus a nocturnal preference (eg, "night owl" or late chronotype). Evidence suggests that matching shift type for individuals with extreme chronotypes (eg, night shifts for those with late chronotype) can be beneficial for sleep and work productivity[37]; however, this may not be commonly feasible across occupational settings. Nonetheless, information about chronotype may predict adaptation to the shift schedule.

Circadian preference can be assessed via clinical assessment or questionnaires validated for shift workers. There are various measures of chronotype, but only the Munich Chronotype Questionnaire for Shift Workers (MCTQShift) is validated for shift workers. The MCTQShift yields a continuous measure of chronotype based on sleep behavior, and has been studied in large representative samples; however, no categorical cutoffs are provided for early versus late chronotypes, although clinical judgment may be made based on the distribution of chronotypes in a representative sample. Information on chronotype may inform intervention strategies (eg, support in adjusting to shift work vs terminating shift work), particularly for individuals with extreme chronotypes.

Circadian Phase

One challenge of clinical management of SWD is the lack of access to information about the biological clock. Although collection of hourly salivary melatonin over a 24-hour period can be used to determine the onset and/or offset of endogenous melatonin (eg, dim light melatonin onset) as an index of circadian phase, this process is presently too resource intensive for clinical feasibility. However, alternative and more efficient methods of approximating circadian phase have become nascent with recent scientific advances. There is preliminary evidence that analyses of gene expression using 2 blood samples taken 12 hours apart can accurately predict circadian phase (82% of predictions were within 2 hours of observed circadian phase).[38] There is also evidence that a single epidermis sample also can produce estimates of circadian phase that are accurate within 3 hours.[39] Finally, preliminary evidence shows that light and activity history in night-shift workers collected passively via actigraphy can lead to accurate estimates within 2 hours of observed dim light melatonin onset.[40] Although promising, these approaches need further validation before they can be integrated into clinical practice.

CLINICAL MANAGEMENT OF SHIFT WORK DISORDER

Approaches to the clinical management of SWD can target symptoms or resolve the potential underlying circadian misalignment. Managing symptoms of sleep-wake disturbances can include both pharmacologic and nonpharmacologic strategies. A stepwise progression is generally recommended, focusing first on improving daytime sleep and then addressing residual complaints of sleepiness or impaired function during the night shift. However, safety always should be prioritized in treatment strategies, as is the case when there are concerns about drowsy driving or other risk of accidents or injuries.

Pharmacologic Interventions

Sleep

For patients who have difficulty initiating daytime sleep at the desired time despite optimal sleep hygiene, a short-acting hypnotic agent can be used to promote daytime sleep[41] (**Table 2**). Meta-analyses of randomized, placebo-controlled trials in patients with insomnia indicate that both benzodiazepines and nonbenzodiazepine receptor agonists improve sleep but have an increased risk of side effects compared with placebo.[42,43] Common side effects of hypnotics can include residual sedation, particularly with sleep periods less than 7 hours, and careful monitoring of potential adverse events is critical in shift workers due to the increased prevalence of excessive sleepiness in this population. The risk of carryover of sedative effects into the night shift should be discussed with individuals who are considering pharmacotherapy, particularly if longer-acting hypnotics are used.

Limited studies in shift workers have demonstrated improvements of 30 to 60 minutes in daytime sleep with use of short-acting nonbenzodiazepines such as zolpidem and short-acting or intermediate-acting benzodiazepines such as triazolam and temazepam.[41,44,45] However, it is important to recognize that use of hypnotics may not eliminate excessive sleepiness, especially in patients with circadian misalignment. In such cases, it may be critical to target the realignment of circadian rhythms to match the sleep-wake schedule using bright artificial light exposure.[46]

Exogenous melatonin also may be used to support daytime sleep in shift workers (use of exogenous melatonin is not recommended for insomnia that is not associated with shift work). A meta-analysis of 7 small randomized trials of melatonin versus placebo in night workers (n = 263) found evidence that exogenously administered melatonin (1–10 mg) improves total sleep time.[47] Importantly, no dose-response association was found dose and sleep duration. When exogenous melatonin is used to promote daytime sleep in shift workers, doses of no more than 1 to 10 mg, taken at or shortly before bed time.[41] Similar to use of hypnotics, use of melatonin may not increase alertness during the night shift, and patients may require additional strategies to maximize circadian adaptation.

Sleepiness
Wake-promoting agents may be prescribed for patients with SWD to target excessive nocturnal sleepiness during the night shift. Modafinil and armodafinil are options approved by the Food and Drug Administration in patients with persistent sleepiness in conjunction with nonpharmacologic measures to improve sleep and alertness. In 2 randomized trials of patients with SWD (n = 572), armodafinil (150 mg taken 30–60 minutes before the night shift) improved subjective sleepiness by 1 point on the Karolinska Sleepiness Scale and improved alertness compared with placebo.[48,49] In a separate small randomized trial, armodafinil also improved performance on a driving simulator compared with placebo.[50] Modest but statistically significant benefits also have been observed with modafinil (200 mg) in shift workers.[51] Together, the effects of modafinil and armodafinil appear to improve alertness during shift work, although the magnitude of benefit varies significantly between individuals. Treatment decisions should be individualized, taking into account the severity of symptoms and the potential consequences of impaired alertness (which frequently vary based on job responsibilities) and the risk of side effects. The most common side effects of modafinil and armodafinil are headache and nausea; postmarketing surveillance studies have reported rare cases of Stevens-Johnson syndrome in association with modafinil.[47]

Caffeine also can be used to enhance alertness during the night shift,[52] although timing of use should consider planned sleep periods to avoid interfering with daytime sleep. As such, caffeine use should typically be limited to the first half of the night shift, and a recommended dose between 250 and 400 mg (~1–4 cups depending on strength). Evidence suggests that single doses of at the beginning of a night shift may be more alerting than divided doses.[53] Caffeine also may be used in combination with a nap during the night shift to counteract sleep inertia on awakening.[54]

Nonpharmacologic Interventions

Sleep
Symptoms of SWD also may be managed with behavioral strategies that target improvement of sleep. A regular sleep schedule that can be followed even during off-work periods is encouraged to promote stability in circadian entrainment. This may need to be individualized, as shift workers often require flexibility to meet varying social and family obligations. Although a consolidated 7 to 8 hours of sleep is recommended, daytime sleep can be separated into 2 bouts to accommodate the need for flexibility: the first, a regularized 3-hour to 4-hour "anchor" sleep that takes priority,

and a second bout that can vary around other responsibilities (total sleep should fall between 7 and 9 hours). Some individuals with SWD may also benefit from an adaptation of cognitive behavioral therapy for insomnia (CBT-I), although this has yet to be tested in a large and well-controlled studies. Adaptations for CBT-I for SWD may focus more on sleep scheduling instead of sleep restriction, and may include use of timed exposure to sunlight or artificial bright light.[55–57]

When possible, the sleep environment should be designed to promote consolidated daytime sleep, with particular attention to light, temperature, and noise level. Light-blocking shades should be used to reduce as much sunlight as possible, with cool ambient temperature (generally between 60 and 75°F). If ambient noise cannot be controlled, a white noise machine may help reduce arousals that are due to variability in environmental noise.

Sleepiness
Multiple studies have indicated that naps before or during the night shift can effectively improve alertness and performance during the shift.[54,58–62] Naps may be planned before the shift or late in the shift to improve alertness and performance. For patients who are symptomatic despite adequate or optimized daytime sleep, behavioral strategies include the use of naps before or during the night shift (recommended <60 minutes), and can be combined with caffeine. For safety critical operations, naps should be limited to less than 60 minutes to minimize the chances of entering deep sleep and to reduce disorientation from sleep inertia on awakening.[63] However, those with more severe sleep deprivation may benefit from arrangements that allow for longer naps with planned time for dissipation of sleep inertia before resuming work.

Circadian realignment
Clinical management of SWD can also aim to resolve the underlying circadian misalignment. This can be achieved either by aligning the work schedule to the biological clock, or resetting the biological clock to synchronize with the nocturnal work schedule. Although some shift workers with SWD have the option of switching to a fixed day-shift schedule, this is often not an option given occupational demands or job availability. Recent evidence also supports matching individuals with extreme chronotypes with work schedules (ie, night shifts for extreme late chronotypes, and morning shifts for extreme morning chronotypes).[37] Although the implementation of this in most occupational settings may be limited, in severe cases, clinicians may choose to provide a letter on the patient's behalf, explaining the disorder and its consequences with the aim of having a patient moved to a day-shift schedule out of medical necessity.

Alternatively, the biological clock also can be shifted to be better aligned with the work schedule using light exposure and/or melatonin. Specifically, timed exposure to bright light (2000–10,000 lux at the retina) has the potential to reduce the mismatch between an individual's internal circadian phase and the desired or environmental schedule, and limited data indicate that such interventions may be useful in shift workers to improve alertness. Light exposure has demonstrated effectiveness at various doses, ranging from as low as four 20-minute periods during breaks to as much exposure during the shift as possible.[41] Light may serve to improve alertness and/or shift circadian rhythms as indexed by the timing of body temperature minimum or melatonin onset. On average, each hour of exposure to bright light can incur a 30-minute shift in the biological clock.

For workers on the night shift, light-blocking glasses used in the morning (approximately 6–11 AM) also can be helpful, especially when shift workers may be exposed to natural sunlight before their scheduled daytime sleep (eg, on the commute home). Similarly, light-blocking shades should be installed in the sleeping environment to prevent exposure to sunlight during daytime sleep.

Table 2
Summary of clinical management strategies to improve sleep and reduce sleepiness

Type	Purpose	Strategy
Pharmacologic	Improve sleep	Hypnotics (benzodiazepines and non-benzodiazepines)
		Exogenous melatonin for daytime sleep
	Reduce sleepiness	Wake-promoting agents (modafinil, armodafinil)
		Caffeine
Nonpharmacological	Improve sleep	Regularized sleep to the extent possible
		Anchor sleep
		Dark, quiet, and cool sleep environment
	Reduce sleepiness	Planned naps
		Caffeine naps
	Circadian alignment	Match extreme chronotypes with respective work shift
		Timed exposure to artificial light
		Timed exposure to darkness (or use of light-blocking glasses)
		Timed use of melatonin as a chronobiotic

Safety

Many shift workers are employed in safety-sensitive or transportation occupations, and excessive sleepiness and accidents should be discussed and monitored throughout treatment. The Epworth Sleepiness Scale can be helpful in tracking risk and response to treatment in a standardized manner. Drowsy driving should be assessed, including any history of vehicular accidents or near-misses attributable to sleepiness, fatigue, or inattention. Behavioral methods of reducing such risks should be reviewed with the patient and with family members, when possible, including the safest option of arranging for a ride home after a night shift. Many occupational settings that employ shift workers (eg, health care systems) provide taxi and other ride-share services as an employee benefit.

SUMMARY

The impact of SWD is varied and far-reaching. As globalization continues, so does the demand for a 24/7 workforce. As such, it is imperative for health care providers to have clinical resources (eg, assessments, effective interventions) that can support shift workers in leading healthy and productive lives. The benefits of a healthy 24/7 workforce reaches public health, as the cascading consequences when occupational safety is compromised can be pervasive (eg, accidents with multiple fatalities, factory error that compromises the environment). The strategies described in this article can support employee health and aid in reducing and preventing accidents, injuries, and fatalities.

REFERENCES

1. Boivin DB, Boudreau P. Impacts of shift work on sleep and circadian rhythms. Pathol Biol 2014;62(5):292–301.
2. Parent-Thirion A, Vermeylen G, van Houten G, et al. Fifth European survey on working conditions. 2014.

3. Cheng P, Drake CL. Psychological impact of shift work. Curr Sleep Med Rep 2018;4(2):104–9.

4. Drake CL, Roehrs T, Richardson G, et al. Shift work sleep disorder: prevalence and consequences beyond that of symptomatic day workers. Sleep 2004; 27(8):1453–62.

5. American Academy of Sleep Medicine. The international classification of sleep disorders: diagnostic and coding manual. Darien (CT): Amercian Academy of Sleep Medicine; 2014.

6. Grundy A, Cotterchio M, Kirsh VA, et al. Rotating shift work associated with obesity in men from northeastern Ontario. Health Promot Chronic Dis Prev Can 2017;37(8):238–47.

7. Bonham MP, Bonnell EK, Huggins CE. Energy intake of shift workers compared to fixed day workers: a systematic review and meta-analysis. Chronobiol Int 2016; 33(8):1086–100.

8. Scheer FAJL, Hilton MF, Mantzoros CS, et al. Adverse metabolic and cardiovascular consequences of circadian misalignment. Proc Natl Acad Sci U S A 2009; 106(11):4453–8.

9. Knutsson A, Kempe A. Shift work and diabetes – a systematic review. Chronobiol Int 2014;31(10):1146–51.

10. Pan A, Schernhammer ES, Sun Q, et al. Rotating night shift work and risk of type 2 diabetes: two prospective cohort studies in women. PLoS Med 2011;8(12): e1001141.

11. Yuan X, Zhu C, Wang M, et al. Night shift work increases the risks of multiple primary cancers in women: a systematic review and meta-analysis of 61 articles. Cancer Epidemiol Biomarkers Prev 2018;27(1):25–40.

12. Li Y, Li S, Zhou Y, et al. Melatonin for the prevention and treatment of cancer. Oncotarget 2017;8(24):39896–921.

13. Reiter RJ, Rosales-Corral SA, Tan D-X, et al. Melatonin, a full service anti-cancer agent: inhibition of initiation, progression and metastasis. Int J Mol Sci 2017;18(4) [pii:E843].

14. Graw P, Kräuchi K, Knoblauch V, Wirz-Justice A, Cajochen C. Circadian and wake-dependent modulation of fastest and slowest reaction times during the psychomotor vigilance task. Physiology & behavior 2004;80(5):695–701.

15. Horowitz TS, Cade BE, Wolfe JM, Czeisler CA. Searching Night and Day A Dissociation of Effects of Circadian Phase and Time Awake on Visual Selective Attention and Vigilance. Psychological Science 2003;14(6):549–57.

16. Van Dongen H, Dinges DF. Sleep, circadian rhythms, and psychomotor vigilance. Clinics in sports medicine 2005;24(2):237–49.

17. Cheng P, Tallent G, Bender TJ, et al. Shift work and cognitive flexibility: decomposing task performance. J Biol Rhythms 2017;32(2):143–53.

18. Belcher R, Gumenyuk V, Roth T. Insomnia in shift work disorder relates to occupational and neurophysiological impairment. J Clin Sleep Med 2015;11(4):457–65.

19. Gumenyuk V, Roth T, Korzyukov O, et al. Shift work sleep disorder is associated with an attenuated brain response of sensory memory and an increased brain response to novelty: an ERP study. Sleep 2010;33(5):703.

20. US Chemical Safety Board. Refinery explosion and fire. Washington, DC: US Chemical Safety Board; 2007.

21. Marquié J-C, Tucker P, Folkard S, et al. Chronic effects of shift work on cognition: findings from the VISAT longitudinal study. Occup Environ Med 2015;72(4):258–64.

22. Monk T, Buysse D, Reynolds C III, et al. Circadian rhythms in human performance and mood under constant conditions. J Sleep Res 1997;6(1):9–18.

23. McClung CA. Circadian genes, rhythms and the biology of mood disorders. Pharmacol Ther 2007;114(2):222–32.
24. Books C, Coody LC, Kauffman R, et al. Night shift work and its health effects on nurses. Health Care Manag 2017;36(4):347–53.
25. Ferri P, Guadi M, Marcheselli L, et al. The impact of shift work on the psychological and physical health of nurses in a general hospital: a comparison between rotating night shifts and day shifts. Risk Manag Healthc Policy 2016;9:203.
26. Angerer P, Schmook R, Elfantel I, et al. Night work and the risk of depression. Dtsch Arztebl Int 2017;114(24):404–11.
27. Kalmbach DA, Pillai V, Cheng P, et al. Shift work disorder, depression, and anxiety in the transition to rotating shifts: the role of sleep reactivity. Sleep Med 2015; 16(12):1532–8.
28. Bildt C, Michélsen H. Gender differences in the effects from working conditions on mental health: a 4-year follow-up. Int Arch Occup Environ Health 2002; 75(4):252–8.
29. Driesen K, Jansen NWH, van Amelsvoort LGPM, et al. The mutual relationship between shift work and depressive complaints - a prospective cohort study. Scand J Work Environ Health 2011;37(5):402–10.
30. Nabe-nielsen K, Garde AH, Albertsen K, et al. The moderating effect of work-time influence on the effect of shift work: a prospective cohort study. Int Arch Occup Environ Health 2011;84(5):551–9.
31. Aldous J. Occupational characteristics and males' role performance in the family. J Marriage Fam 1969;31(4):707–12.
32. Becker L, Barnes M. Understanding participatory time for groups at risk of social exclusion. London, England: Presented at: 2nd Advisory Group Meeting for the National Center for Social Research; 2009.
33. Jensen HI, Larsen JW, Thomsen TD. The impact of shift work on intensive care nurses' lives outside work: a cross-sectional study. J Clin Nurs 2018;27(3–4): e703–9.
34. Bastien CH, Vallières A, Morin CM. Validation of the insomnia severity index as an outcome measure for insomnia research. Sleep Med 2001;2(4):297–307.
35. Chervin RD, Aldrich MS, Pickett R, et al. Comparison of the results of the Epworth sleepiness scale and the multiple sleep latency test. J Psychosom Res 1997; 42(2):145–55.
36. Delafosse J, Léger D, Quera-Salva M, et al. Comparative study of actigraphy and ambulatory polysomnography in the assessment of adaptation to night shift work in nurses. Rev Neurol (Paris) 2000;156(6–7):641–5.
37. Vetter C, Fischer D, Matera JL, et al. Aligning work and circadian time in shift workers improves sleep and reduces circadian disruption. Curr Biol 2015; 25(7):907–11.
38. Laing EE, Möller-Levet CS, Poh N, et al. Blood transcriptome based biomarkers for human circadian phase. Elife 2017;6:e20214.
39. Wu G, Ruben MD, Schmidt RE, et al. Population-level rhythms in human skin with implications for circadian medicine. Proc Natl Acad Sci U S A 2018;115(48): 12313–8.
40. Cheng P, Walch O, Tran K, et al. Using mathematical modeling to preduct circadian phase in night shift workers. In: SLEEP. Vol 41. OXFORD UNIV PRESS INC JOURNALS DEPT, 2001 EVANS RD, CARY, NC 27513 USA; 2018:A237.
41. Morgenthaler T, Lee-Chiong T, Alessi C, et al. Practice parameters for the clinical evaluation and treatment of circadian rhythm sleep disorders: an American Academy of Sleep Medicine report. Sleep 2007;30(11):1445.

42. Buscemi N, Vandermeer B, Friesen C, et al. The efficacy and safety of drug treatments for chronic insomnia in adults: a meta-analysis of RCTs. J Gen Intern Med 2007;22(9):1335.
43. Huedo-Medina TB, Kirsch I, Middlemass J, et al. Effectiveness of non-benzodiazepine hypnotics in treatment of adult insomnia: meta-analysis of data submitted to the Food and Drug Administration. BMJ 2012;345:e8343.
44. Balkin TJ, O'Donnell VM, Wesensten N, et al. Comparison of the daytime sleep and performance effects of zolpidem versus triazolam. Psychopharmacology (Berl) 1992;107(1):83–8.
45. Walsh JK, Schweitzer PK, Anch AM, et al. Sleepiness/alertness on a simulated night shift following sleep at home with triazolam. Sleep 1991;14(2):140–6.
46. Eastman CI, Martin SK. How to use light and dark to produce circadian adaptation to night shift work. Ann Med 1999;31(2):87–98.
47. Liira J, Verbeek J, Ruotsalainen J. Pharmacological interventions for sleepiness and sleep disturbances caused by shift work. JAMA 2015;313(9):961–2.
48. Czeisler CA, Walsh JK, Wesnes KA, et al. Armodafinil for treatment of excessive sleepiness associated with shift work disorder: a randomized controlled study. Mayo Clin Proc 2009;84(11):958–72.
49. Erman MK, Seiden DJ, Yang R, et al. Efficacy and tolerability of armodafinil: effect on clinical condition late in the shift and overall functioning of patients with excessive sleepiness associated with shift work disorder. J Occup Environ Med 2011;53(12):1460.
50. Drake CL, Gumenyuk V, Roth T, et al. Effects of armodafinil on simulated driving and alertness in shift work disorder. Sleep 2014;37(12):1987–94.
51. Czeisler CA, Walsh JK, Roth T, et al. Modafinil for excessive sleepiness associated with shift-work sleep disorder. N Engl J Med 2005;353(5):476–86.
52. Ker K, Edwards PJ, Felix LM, et al. Caffeine for the prevention of injuries and errors in shift workers. Cochrane Database Syst Rev 2010;(5):CD008508.
53. Walsh JK, Muehlbach MJ, Schweitzer PK. Hypnotics and caffeine as countermeasures for shiftwork-related sleepiness and sleep disturbance. J Sleep Res 1995;4:80–3.
54. Schweitzer PK, Randazzo AC, Stone K, et al. Laboratory and field studies of naps and caffeine as practical countermeasures for sleep-wake problems associated with night work. Sleep 2006;29(1):39–50.
55. Eastman CI, Boulos Z, Terman M, et al. Light treatment for sleep disorders: consensus report VI. Shift work. J Biol Rhythms 1995;10(2):157–64.
56. Revell VL, Burgess HJ, Gazda CJ, et al. Advancing human circadian rhythms with afternoon melatonin and morning intermittent bright light. J Clin Endocrinol Metab 2006;91(1):54–9.
57. Zee PC, Goldstein CA. Treatment of shift work disorder and jet lag. Curr Treat Options Neurol 2010;12(5):396–411.
58. Bonnefond A, Muzet A, Winter-Dill A-S, et al. Innovative working schedule: introducing one short nap during the night shift. Ergonomics 2001;44(10):937–45.
59. Chinoy ED, Harris MP, Kim MJ, et al. Scheduled evening sleep and enhanced lighting improve adaptation to night shift work in older adults. Occup Environ Med 2016;73(12):869–76.
60. Garbarino S, Mascialino B, Penco MA, et al. Professional shift-work drivers who adopt prophylactic naps can reduce the risk of car accidents during night work. Sleep 2004;27(7):1295–302.

61. Purnell MT, Feyer A-M, Herbison GP. The impact of a nap opportunity during the night shift on the performance and alertness of 12-h shift workers. J Sleep Res 2002;11(3):219–27.
62. Sallinen M, Härmä M, Åkerstedt T, et al. Promoting alertness with a short nap during a night shift. J Sleep Res 1998;7(4):240–7.
63. Rosekind MR, Gander PH, Gregory KB, et al. Managing fatigue in operational settings 1: physiological considerations and countermeasures. Behav Med 1996; 21(4):157–65.

Challenging Circadian Rhythm Disorder Cases

Melanie Pogach, MD, MMSc, Robert Joseph Thomas, MD, MMSc*

KEYWORDS

- Circadian • Biological night • Actigraphy • Melatonin profile

KEY POINTS

- The classic circadian rhythm disorders have specific criteria and are readily recognizable, but variations to these descriptions are frequent in clinical practice.
- Measurement is key; both actigraphy and melatonin profiling are recommended for accurate diagnosis of classic and nonclassic presentations. Melatonin mapping may be restricted to a portion of the 24-hour period, such as dim-light melatonin onset, or across a full 24 hours, to map the entire biological night.
- Unique challenges in diagnosis and treatment include a long biological night, circadian mechanisms for sleep inertia in idiopathic hypersomnia, iatrogenic hypermelatoninemia, lithium-sensitive cyclical insomnia, electronic media syndrome, mixed physiology (circadian plus), and irregular sleep-wake patterns in severe medical illnesses.
- Treatment of atypical circadian rhythm disorders can pose challenges but can be improved with measurement of circadian biomarkers and personalized circadian-based approaches.

INTRODUCTION

The classic circadian rhythm disorders have discrete diagnostic criteria and are clinically recognizable. However, the circadian system and its interaction with sleep and sleep disorders can result in a large range of patterns that do not quite fit. This finding should not be surprising, because sleep homeostasis affects suprachiasmatic nucleus activity,[1] and circadian gene mutants often have abnormal sleep-wake rhythms.[2–4]

Disclosure: Dr R.J. Thomas is coinventor and patent holder of the ECG-derived sleep spectrogram, which may be used to phenotype sleep quality and central/complex sleep apnea. The technology is licensed by Beth Israel Deaconess Medical Center to MyCardio, LLC. He is also coinventor and patent holder of the Positive Airway Pressure Gas Modulator, being developed for treatment of central/complex sleep apnea. He is a consultant to Jazz Pharmaceuticals and GLG Councils and was a consultant in software development for DeVilbiss-Drive. Dr M. Pogach reports no conflicts and has nothing to declare.
Department of Internal Medicine, Division of Pulmonary, Critical Care and Sleep Medicine, Beth Israel Deaconess Medical Center, KB-23 (Pulmonary Office), 300 Brookline Avenue, Boston, MA 02215, USA
* Corresponding author.
E-mail address: rthomas1@bidmc.harvard.edu

Mutation of the human CRY1 gene can cause familial delayed sleep phase disorder, but sleep is also substantially fragmented.[5] Actigraphy monitoring has been a standard for the diagnosis of circadian rhythm disorders, whereas profiling of internal circadian biomarkers such as melatonin, cortisol, and core body temperature have largely been research tools. Once such testing is routinely used in clinical practice, the spectrum of disorders is likely to expand. The following case-based descriptions provide an early look into some of the less common and challenging abnormalities of circadian rhythms. Because of the limited clinical trial evidence for clinical treatments, in these cases, most of the treatments are empiric, using circadian-based principles.

Case 1: The Long Biological Night Syndrome

Driving mechanisms in idiopathic hypersomnia remain poorly defined. The definition of idiopathic hypersomnia includes showing a total sleep time with unconstrained recordings of 660 minutes or more, and the absence of narcolepsy features including rapid eye movement (REM) pressure phenomena and cataplexy.[6] The traditional polysomnographic testing for evaluating hypersomnia requires a minimum of 6 hours of sleep followed by a next-day multiple sleep latency test (MSLT) to quantify sleep latency (for hypersomnia of any cause) and entry into REM sleep (for narcolepsy).[7] However, this diagnostic model gives little consideration to the total sleep capability of the individual or the positioning of the test in the biological day, both of which present potential confounding of interpretation because of potential encroachment of the biological night into the timing of the early naps of the MSLT.[7] Results of the MSLT in narcolepsy type I are stable over time, whereas it is not for narcolepsy type II[8] or idiopathic hypersomnia.[9,10] The authors measure the biological night in patients with clinical presentations consistent with idiopathic hypersomnia, which has shown that most (>80 tested) of those with long sleep also have a long biological night.

The case described here is a 34-year old woman with idiopathic hypersomnia (polysomnogram total sleep time 11 hours and 52 minutes, sleep log average total sleep time 12.6 hours). Sleep inertia is severe, and there is no cataplexy or depression. Polysomnography showed a total sleep time of 711 minutes. She is on no medications other than oral contraceptives. She works 5 days a week from 8 AM to 6:30 PM, and wakes up at 7 AM; bedtime is 10 PM; on the weekend, she sleeps until 12 noon or beyond. A 24-hour salivary melatonin mapping was done (**Fig. 1**).

A circadian mechanism for idiopathic hypersomnia was recently described[11] in a study comparing fibroblasts from skin biopsies of patients with idiopathic hypersomnia and healthy subjects. The circadian period length of the primary fibroblast cells was determined by lentiviral infection with a construct expressing a luciferase gene under the control of a BMAL1 promoter. Compared with the group of healthy controls, the mean period length of patients with idiopathic hypersomnia was estimated to be 0.82 hours (95% confidence interval, 0.44–1.20 hours) longer in the patient group. The amplitude of the rhythmically expressed BMAL1, PER1, and PER2 has been reportedly dampened in dermal fibroblasts of idiopathic hypersomnia compared with healthy controls, and the overall expression of BMAL1 was reduced.[12] A longer circadian period may contribute to hypersomnia if associated with a lower amplitude of the circadian alertness drive in the morning, and may be a mechanism for the severe sleep inertia that characterizes idiopathic hypersomnia with long sleep time. Delayed phase has been reported in patients with idiopathic hypersomnia.[13]

Diagnostic challenges

An established long biological night, as measured by prolonged increase of melatonin profiles, including living in the polar extremes,[14,15] seasonal affective

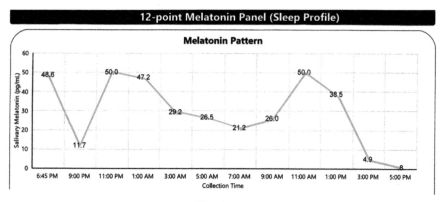

Fig. 1. A 24-hour salivary melatonin profile. The test is performed at home, under less than 10-lux light established using the Light Meter phone application (https://play.google.com/store/apps/details?id=com.tsang.alan.lightmeter&hl=en_US). This profile is an example of a long biological night. Only 1 of the 12 samples, measured every 2 hours, is within the accepted norm of 3 pg/mL.

disorder during the winter months,[16] and the blind.[17] The biological night also expands in healthy persons exposed to natural outdoor winter.[18] Habitual long sleepers have a longer biological night than habitual short sleepers.[19] A common genetic variant in a receptor for the circadian-regulated hormone melatonin (MTNR1B) is associated with increased fasting blood glucose level and risk of type 2 diabetes mellitus. However, there is also a substantially longer duration of increased melatonin levels (41 minutes) and delayed circadian phase of dim-light melatonin onset (1.37 hours) in people with this variant, partially mediated through delayed onset of melatonin synthesis.[20] The authors do not have genomic analysis in our patients, but similar mechanisms could be important.

Those who currently receive a diagnosis of narcolepsy without cataplexy (type II narcolepsy) and who are able to sleep for long durations could be considered possible false-positives because the early naps of typical MSLTs are timed partially in the biological night. This confounding effect of testing in the biological night may explain in part the inconsistency of repeat MSLTs in type II versus type I narcolepsy[9,21]; a patient with idiopathic hypersomnia may fit narcolepsy type II on one testing occasion and not on another.

Treatment challenges
Stimulant may be less likely to be effective when used in the biological night and may explain some of the variability in clinical response to these agents.[22,23] A further option could be using β-blockers to reduce melatonin levels, as has been evaluated in seasonal affective disorder.[24,25]

Treatment plan
This patient has responded clinically to propranolol, 10 mg at 7 AM and 3 PM, with a reduction of sleep duration capability from 14 to 15 hours to 7 to 8 hours, Epworth Sleepiness Scale moved from 14 to 8, and daytime fatigue was very much improved. Stimulants were added with additional benefit. Use of β-blockers for idiopathic hypersomnia associated with a long biological night will need substantial new data before generalized use.

Case 2: A Mechanism of Sleep Inertia in Idiopathic Hypersomnia

A 30-year old woman with idiopathic hypersomnia complained of a persistent inability to motivate herself for any task for the first 3 to 4 hours after awakening (natural, about 8 AM). Associated medical conditions include fibromyalgia, inappropriate sinus tachycardia, postural orthostatic tachycardia, and chronic fatigue syndrome. Salivary melatonin testing **(Fig. 2)** was performed immediately after awakening. Bright light therapy on awakening has not had benefit.

Diagnostic challenges
Sleep inertia is a particularly difficult problem to diagnose and treat in patients with idiopathic hypersomnia. Sodium oxybate has reportedly been of benefit.[26] If the mechanism is circadian, bright light or even β-blockers, which can reduce melatonin level[27,28] and even suppress hypermelatoninemia,[29,30] could be a therapeutic option.

Treatment challenges
Long-sleeping patients with idiopathic hypersomnia may see improvements in sleep inertia with the use of sodium oxybate. Bright light, caffeine, amphetamine-based stimulants, exercise, a cold shower, and nicotine are options patients variously use.

Treatment plan
Bright light on awakening and low-dose β-blockers are plausible options, but neither was effective in this patient. β-Blockers can reduce melatonin levels, but therapeutic use of this effect has been difficult.

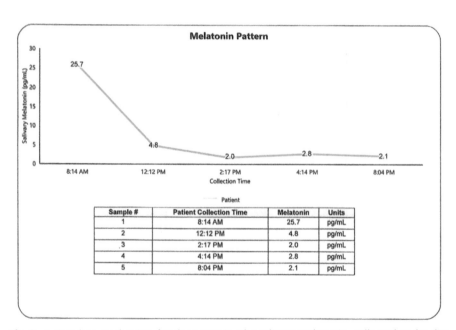

Melatonin Pattern

Sample #	Patient Collection Time	Melatonin	Units
1	8:14 AM	25.7	pg/mL
2	12:12 PM	4.8	pg/mL
3	2:17 PM	2.0	pg/mL
4	4:14 PM	2.8	pg/mL
5	8:04 PM	2.1	pg/mL

Fig. 2. A circadian mechanism for sleep inertia. The salivary melatonin, collected under dim light conditions (less than 10 lux) shows a marked increase of melatonin level at 25.7 pg/mL at the time of awakening, mildly increased around the time of resolution of sleep inertia, and then normal values until the late evening.

Case 3: Boarding School Syndrome

A 16-year old with delayed sleep-wake phase disorder (typical bedtime 2–3 AM, natural wake time 12–1 AM) presents with severe daytime sleepiness and fragmentation of the sleep-wake cycle, with naps in the day, falling asleep in class, and at risk of dismissal from a boarding school. The school has a strict 3-strikes-and-out policy for late class arrival. Wake time is enforced at 6 AM, classes start at 8 AM. Until the imposition of the strict boarding school time protocols, the patient simply missed or was late for classes. There was progressive delay of sleep to nearly 4 AM, extreme inertia on awakening, falling asleep in classes, and long afternoon naps. The Actigraph shown in **Fig. 3** was performed after taking a leave from school, in the home environment.

Diagnostic challenges

The simple delayed pattern has evolved into a far more irregular pattern. There are long wake periods and estimated sleep periods of variable duration. Presumably there was variably timed light exposure in light-sensitive portions of the phase-response curve from the enforced awakenings, which resulted in loss of circadian-sleep synchrony. The patient is not helping his case by keeping the lights on until the very edge of the wake period.

Treatment challenges

Treatment of delayed sleep-wake phase disorder requires timed light exposure after the end of the biological night.[31] Simply and abruptly enforcing a very early wake time does not typically solve the circadian delay and may cause harm by inducing a more fragmented and dysregulated pattern.

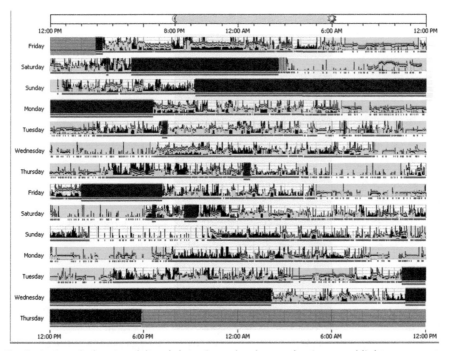

Fig. 3. Actigraph showing delayed sleep, irregular sleep-wake times, and light exposure to the edge of sleep. Blue periods are excluded data, presumably wrist-off time.

Treatment plan

This patient returned to his "normal" delay pattern by keeping a 12-hour light/dark cycle with a "dawn" at 3 PM Ultimately, correction of circadian phase will require the patient to want to make the change.

Case 4: Cirrhosis and Sleep

A 56-year old man with hepatic cirrhosis from alcohol and hepatitis C virus infection presents with insomnia. He uses oral lactulose for mild hepatic encephalopathy. He describes absence of a predictable sleep pattern. Low-dose melatonin (0.15 mg) at 10 PM caused sedation and disorientation and was thus discontinued. Bright light therapy was recommended as part of maintaining a strong light/dark cycle, but the patient was unable to follow recommendations. The actigraphic recording is shown in **Fig. 4**, revealing the loss of a discernible sleep-wake rhythm.

Disruption of the sleep-wake cycle is a well-known feature of advanced cirrhosis[32–34] and is seen in experimental models of portacaval shunts.[35,36] Melatonin metabolism is impaired by liver disease, which could be part of the explanation for abnormal sleep-wake rhythms.[37] Patients with cirrhosis have markedly increased melatonin levels during daytime hours and an overall delay pattern.[38,39] Treatment is difficult, because sedatives are generally contraindicated, and melatonin may not be effective because of already existing hypermelatoninemia. Light therapy may be beneficial, but no trials have been reported.

Diagnostic challenges

Both insomnia and hypersomnia can occur and coexist in advanced liver disease, especially cirrhosis. Worsening sleep can also be a feature of impending

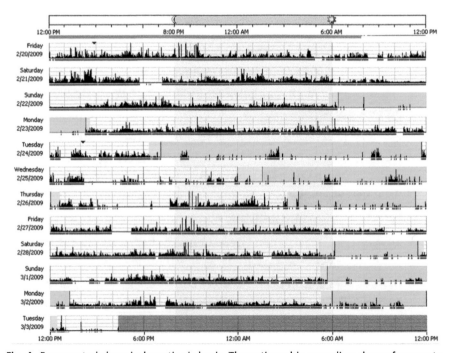

Fig. 4. Fragmented sleep in hepatic cirrhosis. The actigraphic recording shows fragmentation of the sleep-wake cycle, with prolonged activity periods and variable sleep times. Most sleep occurs in a delayed, nearly inverted pattern.

encephalopathy. Melatonin profiles are delayed in cirrhosis. A delayed pattern of sleep-wake can degenerate into an irregular sleep-wake pattern. Thus, accurate characterization of the sleep disorder may not be possible and can change over days and weeks.

Treatment challenges
Sleep-wake dysregulation interacts with liver function to cause instability of sleep patterns. This dynamism is a challenge and management needs to be individualized.

Treatment plan
Optimizing therapy for hepatic encephalopathy, strong and steady light/dark cycle, and correction of severe phase delay if present are useful strategies. Sedatives should be avoided. Melatonin may not be adequately metabolized in advanced liver disease and is best avoided.

Case 5: Pituitary Apoplexy and Sleep-Wake Cycles

A 70-year old presents with a no clear sleep-wake cycle. She is completely unable to designate a sleep and wake time, maintain a sleep log, or follow light/dark instructions. In 2007, she had a pituitary apoplexy and macroadenoma resection. She complains of unexplained falls, and MRI shows mild cerebellar atrophy. An actigraph is shown in **Fig. 5**, and the stable MRI (repeated serially) in **Fig. 6**.

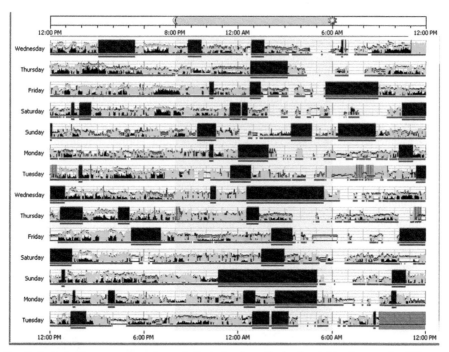

Fig. 5. Postpituitary apoplexy sleep. Actigraphy shows lack of a stable sleep-wake differentiation, although overall activity and light are reduced from just after midnight to 7 to 8 AM. The default algorithms of activity monitors are typically validated against healthy individuals and are not likely to perform well in those with atypical patterns. Note periods of light during the "night," because the patient wakes up frequently. Blue periods are device-off times.

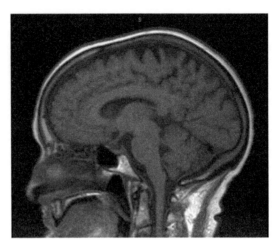

Fig. 6. Pituitary apoplexy. Stable postoperative neuroanatomy.

Diagnostic challenges
Sleep logs and actigraphy alone cannot establish biological day or night when the pattern is so fragmented. Melatonin and ideally melatonin and cortisol profiling are necessary.

Treatment challenges
An important challenge is to establish a structured environment and stable sleep-wake cycle, because instability begets instability.

Treatment plan
A reasonable initial strategy would be to establish a sleep-free zone in the local day, and then use bright light during the wake period, low light and darkness in a prescribed rest period, expanding the light-dark cycle over several weeks to a 12-hour light/dark cycle. Melatonin can be used to create a biological night. Further movement of sleep times will need to be individualized. A daytime stimulant can help maintain a stable wake zone. Secondary narcolepsy, if present, should be treated.

Key Challenge
Abnormal circadian rest-activity and temperature rhythms can occur after lesions in the region of the hypothalamus.[40–42] If the suprachiasmatic nucleus is itself injured, entrainment may be impossible with light-dark cues, but in principle may be possible with feeding, enforced activity, and social cues.

Case 6: Lithium-responsive Cyclical Insomnia
A 52-year old man with attention-deficit/hyperactivity disorder, high loop gain sleep apnea (treated with oral appliance plus 125 mg of acetazolamide) has persistent insomnia. The main feature is wide night-to-night variation of sleep durations. A cyclical pattern is suspected and actigraphy is performed, which confirms it (**Fig. 7**). He has already failed treatment with melatonin, benzodiazepines, sedative antipsychotics, and antihistamines. There was no mood instability, but he did note marked worsening of fatigue following nights with reduced sleep. Because of the similarity of the sleep pattern to mood fluctuations in bipolar disease, a trial of low-dose lithium

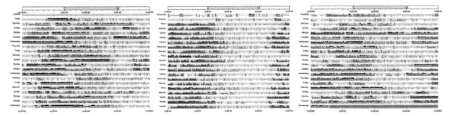

Fig. 7. Lithium-sensitive insomnia. From left: prelithium, while on lithium, and after discontinuation of lithium. Note a clear increase in stability of sleep-wake times and pattern when taking lithium (only 150 mg/day). Activity intensity is also increased while on lithium (the thresholds for the graphs are the same for all 3 components).

was initiated, followed by actigraphic tracking. The patient self-discontinued the medication to confirm for himself the benefits of the drug.

Diagnostic challenges

Insomnia is a heterogeneous condition, and a common symptom in several psychiatric disorders. Bipolar disease is characterized by both sleep and mood instability and is strongly related to abnormal circadian regulation.[43,44] High-risk individuals report irregularity of sleep-wake times, poor sleep, and circadian rhythm disruption.[45] However, the patient described here has never had mood symptoms or features of mania/hypomania, only unstable sleep durations. The worse daytime fatigue associated with short sleep is also the inverse of that noted in mania/hypomania. Cellular clock dysfunction may be common in mood disorders.[46] Lithium is a drug with strong circadian effects[47,48] in humans, and it stabilizes sleep-wake rhythm in the manialike CLOCK mutant mouse.[49,50]

Treatment challenges

Chronic insomnia disorder has well-defined criteria. One component that is not currently considered is the degree of variability of sleep timings and durations. Although mild to moderate night-to-night variability can be expected, severe variability to the extent of completely sleepless nights occurring cyclically should raise the possibility of hypomania. However, a subset of patients have stable mood and unstable sleep, and a cyclic insomnia pattern, and these are characteristically mixed with periods of normal sleep. Actigraphy and sleep logs can capture the variability. Clinical criteria for hypomania are absent, and such patients typically fail cognitive behavior therapy, antidepressants, and sedatives.

Treatment plan

If insomnia is primarily characterized by unstable sleep-wake durations, a trial of low-dose lithium may be beneficial; this discovery was serendipitous in our center. However, lithium seems to have benefits in cyclical disorders, including mania, Kleine-Levin syndrome of cyclical hypersomnia, and cluster headaches, suggesting effects on shared biological pathways.

Case 7: Iatrogenic hypermelatoninemia

A 60-year old woman with lifelong severe delayed sleep-wake phase disorder, has a typical bedtime of 5 to 6 AM. Bedtime melatonin 1 mg hypnotic dose at 4 AM results in improved sleep initiation but more sleep inertia. Melatonin measurements from saliva are done (**Table 1**) on and off the hypnotic dose of melatonin, because there is a concern that the melatonin is worsening sleep inertia.

Chronobiotic (4–5 hours before bedtime) and hypnotic (at bedtime) use of melatonin can have clinical benefit. However, melatonin itself may contribute to sleep inertia, especially if high doses (3–5 mg) or sustained release formulations are used, or there is slow hepatic metabolism. Measurement of melatonin (saliva) after natural awakening is simple and can establish whether melatonin is a possible contributor.

Diagnostic challenges
Sleep inertia is a common problem in delayed sleep-wake phase disorder, sleep deprivation, and idiopathic hypersomnia. Iatrogenic melatonin effects are not usually considered. Some patients present using very high doses (>30 mg), and the risk of persistent hypermelatoninemia (on awakening) is real. Although the dose used here was small, only direct testing can establish a role for melatonin in any hangover effect.

Treatment challenges
Without knowing whether there is hypermelatoninemia (iatrogenic), a morning stimulant is likely to be started, which would be the wrong option in this instance.

Treatment plan
The hypnotic dose of melatonin has to be discontinued, even though there was consequently some difficulty in sleep initiation.

Table 1 Iatrogenic hypermelatoninemia	
Sample 1	331.4 pg/mL
Sample 2	257.3 pg/mL
Sample 3	189.7 pg/mL
12:00 PM	0.01 pg/mL
1:00 PM	3.1 pg/mL
2:00 PM	2.5 pg/mL

Samples 1 to 3 are salivary melatonin samples at noon, 1, and 2 PM after the usual 1-mg bedtime dose of melatonin. All values are strikingly high. Repeat testing after discontinuation of the melatonin shows a return to normal levels.

Case 8: Possible Internal Desynchrony

A 56-year old man presents with lifelong refractory depression, comorbid obsessive-compulsive disorder, anxiety, irregular mood swings subthreshold to mania, and complex sleep apnea. Sleep timings are irregular (onsets 8 PM to 2 AM, offsets 3 AM to 10 AM), and he can fall into irregular sleep-wake spontaneously. He often seems to be phase delayed. Dim-light melatonin onset (DLMO) immediately following a night when he fell asleep at 8 PM and woke up at 4 AM is shown in **Table 2**.

Diagnostic challenges
Circadian dysregulation occurs in depression and especially mania. However, these changes are poorly characterized because the typical circadian protocols (forced desynchrony, constant routine) would be considered too stressful for depressed or manic patients. Thus, clinical (logs) and actigraphic estimates are typical compromises. Persistent internal circadian misalignment plausibly impairs mood and causes depressive symptoms, and this should be suspected especially when sleep-wake timings are irregular. Ideally, both melatonin and cortisol should be mapped in such individuals and correlated/aligned with simultaneous actigraphy.

Table 2	
Internal desynchrony	
8:22 PM	0.4 mg/mL
9:20 PM	1.5
10:15 PM	2.0
11:21 PM	2.0
12:15 AM	3.1
1:12 AM	11.5
2:08 AM	11.2

The DLMO is between 12 midnight and 1 AM, but the patient had initiated sleep at 8 PM the previous night, several hours earlier than anticipated.

Treatment challenges

In this case, DLMO was delayed, but sleep occurred early and out of phase. Melatonin in the late evening can be used to advance circadian phase, along with strict avoidance of light at phase-disrupting times. Behavioral delay of bedtime to better match circadian phase should be attempted but can be difficult if homeostatic drive is displaced to earlier in the local day.

Assumptions are made about internal alignment of sleep and circadian rhythms in clinical practice and research when direct measurements are not made. These assumptions guide empiric use of light and melatonin for therapy. However, as this case shows, substantial internal misalignment (between sleep and circadian rhythms) can be present. The authors do not know whether there are misalignments in other body rhythms in this patient. Some variability of sleep and circadian set-point has also been reported in clinically typical delayed sleep-wake phase disorder.[51,52]

Treatment plan

In this case, melatonin (8 PM) and light (10 AM) have partially stabilized sleep timings. Light therapy can induce hypomania and may be best avoided early in the course of management of circadian rhythm disorders in individuals with hypomanic features.

Case 9: Severe Medical Condition and Irregular Sleep-Wake Patterns

A 67-year old man with severe congestive heart failure (ejection fraction 10%) and Cheyne-Stokes respiration is unable to use positive pressure therapy along with supplemental oxygen. He uses zolpidem to aid in sleep consolidation. He states that he has had no real sleep time for several years. He is admitted for heart failure exacerbation 3 to 4 times a year, each hospitalization lasting about a week, despite tolerable goal-directed heart failure medical therapy. An actigraphic examination is performed (**Fig. 8**).

Diagnostic challenges

Sleep is often severely fragmented in advanced heart failure. This fragmentation goes beyond sleep apnea and may reflect neurohumoral activation at the brainstem/hypothalamic level. When fragmentation is coupled with dispersion of homeostatic sleep drive with napping, a completely irregular pattern can emerge, and may be sustained indefinitely. Melatonin profiling can establish circadian phase, but sleep remains fragile and difficult to manipulate.

Treatment challenges

Fragmentation of the rest-activity cycle can occur with severe medical illnesses, including heart failure.[53] Rest-activity rhythms may have prognostic value in heart

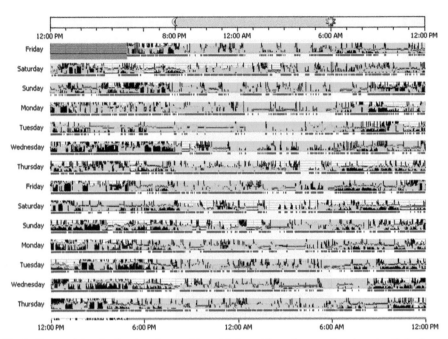

Fig. 8. Rest-activity rhythm in advanced heart failure. There is overall reduced activity from about 8 PM to 8 AM, with substantial variability, increased activity during the sleep period, and substantial light exposure during the local dark period. The estimate of sleep (turquoise periods) is only approximate when sleep-wake activity is so fragmented.

failure.[54,55] In this case, heart failure is severe, as is sleep apnea, coupled with repeated hospitalizations; the hospitalizations are likely a sleep and circadian stressor. Both sleep (apnea and sleep itself) and circadian components need targeting.

Treatment plan

The first step was to define a no-sleep zone, a zone of forced wakefulness in the local day of 3 hours. The next step was to use bright light at both edges of this zone and then move both edges out asymmetrically to target first a 10 PM to 8 AM time zone. Supplemental oxygen was used to reduce periodic breathing, and a sedative (temazepam, 10 PM) was added to consolidate sleep (zolpidem failed). Subsequently, the wake-up time was slowly moved to 6 AM. A rehospitalization disrupted the final part of the plan and, by the time the patient was discharged, the original irregular pattern had returned.

Case 10: Electronic Media Syndrome

A 26-year old woman presents with sleep onset insomnia. She gets into bed around 9 PM but uses various electronic media until 11 PM, and then has difficulty falling asleep until 12 midnight to 1 AM. Wake time is 6 AM on weekdays and 8 AM on weekends. There is daytime fatigue and a midafternoon dip in alertness. A dim-light melatonin test was performed and is shown in **Table 3**.

Diagnostic challenges

Knowing the true circadian phase can be difficult if there is substantial late-night electronic media use.

| Table 3 | | | |
| Electronic device suppression of melatonin | | | |
Sample	Time	pg/mL	Device
1	7:30 PM	2.1	—
2	8:30 PM	13.0	—
3	9:30 PM	3.2	iPAD
4	10:30 PM	2.6	iPAD
5	11:30 PM	4.3	iPAD

During the DLMO testing, the patient "forgot" the instructions to avoid electronic media and used the iPAD in the darkness. Melatonin suppression occurs with use of this electronic device. The background lighting condition from the device is uncertain.

Treatment challenges
Electronic media use in bed is here to stay.[56,57] Mitigation is the key, with technological components (the background lighting, blue filter, intensity), and more research is needed to know what device and setting can and cannot suppress melatonin. Whether there are other alerting effects of light dissociated from melatonin suppression is not known.

Treatment plan
Low-dose melatonin (0.3 mg) at 8 PM and turning down the light intensity to minimal was effective in management. General light hygiene instructions were also provided, and education about phase shifting effects of light.

Case 11: Electronic Media/Light-enhanced Non–24-hour Sleep-Wake Cycle Disorder
A 16-year old with severe delayed sleep-wake phase disorder now has a non–24-hour pattern. Actigraphy is performed (**Fig. 9**). Severe delayed sleep-wake phase disorder can convert into a non–24-hour sleep-wake cycle disorder. In this instance, the constant and stubborn use of electronic media right up to bedtime likely contributed to maintaining the pattern. Behavioral modification is difficult but necessary to stabilize circadian phase in these instances. It is unlikely that melatonin supplementation can stabilize circadian phase when late light exposure is also present.

Diagnostic challenges
Individuals with a tendency to severe circadian phase delay may convert into a non–24-hour pattern by persistent late-night light exposure, especially from electronic devices. Once the pattern is established, it can self-sustain for long periods of time. Exposure to light during the biological night, when mismatched with local time, can accelerate delay or fragment sleep, causing the pattern to become even more interrupted.

Treatment challenges
Demanding an individual entirely stop using late-night electronic media is often unrealistic, but a light curfew is needed to succeed in stabilizing this pattern. Using technology (blue filters in devices, intensity adjustment) can aid in minimizing light driving of delay. Low-dose melatonin (0.3–0.5 mg) can counter the effect of mild increases in evening light. Bright light at the leading end of sleep can slow and eventually stop the clock. After stabilization, adjusting melatonin/light times to align sleep and circadian phase to the desired time can be done over a period of 2 to 3 weeks. The circadian

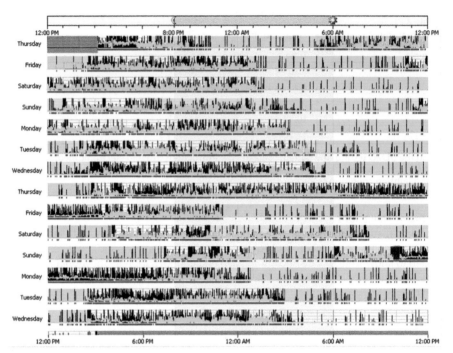

Fig. 9. Electronic media and non–24-hour disorder. Note light exposure (and use of electronic media) right up to sleep time on most nights. Thus, the light exposure also has a progressive pattern across multiple days.

system that has gone around the clock remains vulnerable "for a relapse," at least over the short intermediate term.

Treatment plan

Morning light, evening melatonin, minimizing electronic media, and a curfew (no light after a prespecified time) were used to entrain this patient to a stable but delayed phase. Further phase advance was recommended but not successful, in part because of a return to using late-night iPad-based entertainment.

Case 12 A and B: Advanced Sleep Phase With and Without Comorbidities

Patient A

The first patient is a 73-year-old woman with a body mass index of 20 kg/m², coronary artery disease after stenting, Prinzmetal angina, and atrial fibrillation following ablation, who presented for evaluation of insomnia. Historically, the patient has always been an early riser. Her habitual sleep times range from 9 PM to 4 to 5 AM. She has taken zolpidem for many years. Recently, despite use of zolpidem, she has been waking at 3 to 3:30 AM. There is no napping or inappropriate dozing. Although she feels sleepy in the evenings and could easily fall asleep before 9 PM, she avoids doing so to prevent waking even earlier. Her bedroom is dark, with room-darkening shades. Her living space has few windows and does not capture much daytime sunlight.

A diagnostic polysomnogram was conducted between 10:11 PM and 5:02 AM and showed a pattern suggestive of advanced sleep phase syndrome, exacerbated by first-night effect. The sleep efficiency was reduced to 25.2%. Sleep was fragmented with mostly wake captured after 3:00 AM The apnea-hypopnea index (AHI; 4%) was 0.0 events/h, AHI (AHI 3% or arousal) was 12.75 events/h, the respiratory disturbance index (RDI) was 52 events/h, and the O_2 saturation nadir was 88%. There were no scored periodic limb movements. To guide therapeutic recommendations, salivary melatonin testing was pursued to map the start of the biological night (**Fig. 10**).

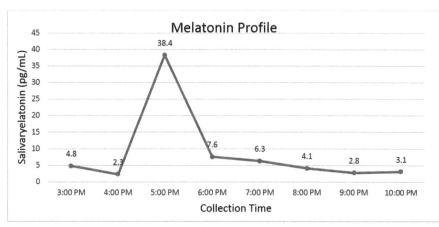

Fig. 10. Advanced salivary melatonin profile. The test was performed in the patient's home, under less than 10-lux light (using Light Meter phone application). The surge in melatonin level, observed between 4 and 5 PM, establishes the early DLMO time. The duration of the surge is short, and, speculatively, it may contribute to short sleep.

Patient B

A healthy 17-year-old woman presented for the evaluation of sleep maintenance insomnia, which became notable following her participation in a computer programming class in high school. Before the course, she did not have sleep problems. Persisting after completion of the course, her sleep remained disrupted by awakenings and her sleep times became dysregulated. She took no medications. Her body mass index was within the normal range at 21 kg/m^2. There were no symptoms suggestive of mood disorder. Her reported sleep schedule varied night to night, with bedtime between 8 and 10 PM on some nights, and from 11 PM to 12 AM on others. She would typically awaken at 2 to 3 AM with difficulty resuming sleep, often using the computer at that time. As her sleep became more disrupted, she began taking naps between 7 and 10 AM and/or in afternoons (weekends 1–3 PM or after school from 4–6 PM).

Her work-up included actigraphy plus sleep logs, which revealed a very irregular sleep-wake cycle; extended polysomnographic recording (recorded from 9:43 PM to 3:00 PM), without evidence of sleep-disordered breathing (AHI 4% of 0.4 events/h and RDI of 7.5 events/h) or periodic limb movements disrupting sleep, with normal sleep and REM latencies, although REM sleep was also observed in the afternoon during extended recording. Salivary DLMO testing was conducted (**Fig. 11**) and showed her melatonin peak at approximately 07:00 PM, suggesting a mild advanced sleep phase. This case is an example of the circadian phase and clinical sleep times (and sleep physiology itself; note that REM sleep occurred after 12 noon during polysomnography) being misaligned, suggesting internal desynchronization.

Insomnia can be both a primary sleep disorder and a symptom of a comorbid sleep disorder, such as a circadian rhythm sleep disorder. Although there are many research tools used to determine circadian rhythms, in the clinical realm available diagnostic

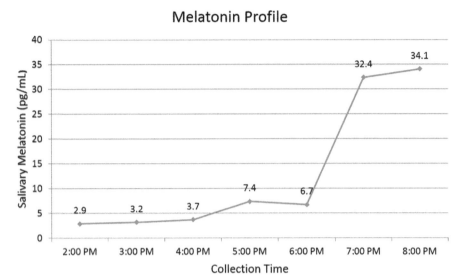

Fig. 11. Salivary melatonin profile. The test was performed in patient's home, under less than 10-lux light (using Light Meter phone application). The surge in melatonin level, observed at the 7 PM time point, establishes the DLMO time.

tests are more limited. In most clinics, and as recommended in current American Academy of Sleep Medicine clinical guidelines, actigraphy and sleep logs are typically used.[26,48] The first patient's clinical history is highly suggestive of advanced sleep phase pattern. Her dark home environment likely contributed to her phase advance, caused by insufficient daytime light exposure. However, melatonin profiling allowed accurate assessment of the onset of her biological night, which allowed effective timing for phototherapy. The sleep patterns of the second patient were more difficult to classify, because she reported very irregular sleep-wake times. Poor sleep habits with device use at night and frequent daytime napping complicated the clinical picture. Initial concerns included phase delay and/or short sleeper. Melatonin sampling was the key to securing an accurate diagnosis and guiding management. The sleep and circadian systems are plastic and fluid, and highly abnormal patterns can be reversed by optimal light/dark cuing and strengthening.

Diagnostic challenges
Whenever an insomniac has less difficulty falling asleep and then early morning awakenings, phase advance is suggested. Over time, interaction of circadian phase with abnormal light exposure, napping, and irregular sleep times can create a chaotic pattern, which then needs a step back and assessment of core sleep and circadian features (melatonin profile, unconstrained polysomnography) to determine therapeutic targets.

Treatment challenges
Patients with substantially advanced phase usually go to bed past their natural bedtimes, guaranteeing early awakening and light/fragmented sleep during the second half of the night. Over-the-counter use of melatonin can worsen phase advance, whereas sedatives in general do not enable consolidated sleep when circadian drive is increasing. When sleep apnea coexists, the second part of sleep may have substantial residual apnea caused by light sleep interacting with positive airway pressure, and

sleep-wake transitions. If a phase abnormality is a key driver of apparent irregular sleep-wake pattern, guiding sleep to the determined phase and then moving that phase to a more desirable time zone is our preferred management approach.

Treatment plan
The treatment plan for advanced sleep phase requires tightening sleep boundaries (consistent bedtimes and wake times) and circadian strategies using strong light and dark cueing with evening phototherapy, avoidance of light/device exposures before and during the desired night zone, and reduction of naps. Melatonin on first awakening can be considered but has a risk of sedation. Tight prescribed sleep times/boundaries and stepwise movement of the same are often required to consolidate sleep and align with circadian phase.

Case 13: Obstructive Sleep Apnea Complicated by Shift Work Disorder

A 51-year-old man with obesity, hypertension, type II diabetes mellitus, and generalized seizure disorder presented after being diagnosed with severe obstructive sleep apnea (AHI 4% of 20 events/h, AHI 3% of 27 events/h, and O_2 nadir of 66%, 76 minutes $\leq 88\%$). He had been initiated on autotitrating continuous positive airway pressure (APAP) set at 8 to 15 cm H_2O but had been unable to meet his insurance usage requirement for ongoing treatment coverage. The patient reported excellent tolerance of APAP with improvement in sleep continuity, resolution of snoring, and increased daytime energy. He used APAP across his sleep whenever he slept at home. However, his average usage was limited by his overnight shift work and frequent overtime, during which he was not able to use APAP. Despite a historical tendency toward a lark chronotype, he has spent years working an overnight shift (10 PM to 6 AM) Sunday to Thursday plus overtime (staying beyond his shift until 12–2 PM) on 2 to 3 of his work days. After work, unless working overtime, he sleeps from 6:30/7 AM until 11 AM to 12 PM (waking spontaneously and feeling refreshed). On off days, he maintains a local nighttime sleep schedule and sleeps well through the night (9 or 10 PM to 6 or 7 AM). **Fig. 12** shows the on and off day sleep schedules.

Diagnostic challenges
When a shift-worker uses continuous positive airway pressure, identifying the cause of residual symptoms can be a challenge. Besides circadian misalignment, total sleep

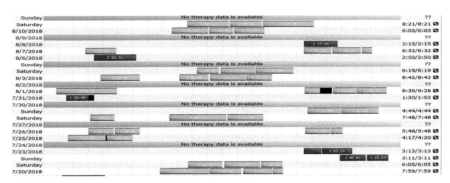

Fig. 12. APAP use in the setting of circadian dysregulation from shift work. APAP use pattern from EncoreAnywhere shows use during daytime sleep after overnight shifts, occasional late naps, following overnights combined with overtime hours, and local time zone sleep on nonwork nights.

time may be reduced, enough to be identified as being noncompliant by insurance coverage criteria.

Treatment challenges

This case shows several clinical care challenges. (1) The patient lives in a state of chronic circadian mismatch, working overnights despite his intrinsic sleep zone remaining on a local sleep schedule. He also has chronic insufficient sleep as a result of his shift work schedule. There is strong evidence from animal, experimental, and epidemiologic studies that insufficient sleep and circadian mismatch contribute to multisystem disorders, including impairments in glucose tolerance, obesity, cardiovascular disease, and malignancy.[58–64]

Treatment plan

Ideally, curtailing shift work would be the most beneficial, but changing the work schedule was not an option. A defined time for sleep on most days of the week was recommended. Longer CPAP use to target minimum insurance requirements is a pragmatic need. Despite suboptimal average sleep duration and circadian misalignment, the patient denied excessive daytime sleepiness and wake-promoting medications have not been needed.

SUMMARY

The cases described here show the range of circadian rhythm abnormalities that can occur in clinical practice far beyond the patterns of the classic circadian rhythm disorders. The paucity of circadian therapies makes management difficult. However, measurement (actigraphy, melatonin profilometry, unconstrained polysomnography) is critical in identifying patterns and therapeutic targets.

REFERENCES

1. Borbely AA, Daan S, Wirz-Justice A, et al. The two-process model of sleep regulation: a reappraisal. J Sleep Res 2016;25(2):131–43.
2. Jagannath A, Taylor L, Wakaf Z, et al. The genetics of circadian rhythms, sleep and health. Hum Mol Genet 2017;26(R2):R128–38.
3. Laposky A, Easton A, Dugovic C, et al. Deletion of the mammalian circadian clock gene BMAL1/Mop3 alters baseline sleep architecture and the response to sleep deprivation. Sleep 2005;28(4):395–409.
4. Wisor JP, O'Hara BF, Terao A, et al. A role for cryptochromes in sleep regulation. BMC Neurosci 2002;3:20.
5. Patke A, Murphy PJ, Onat OE, et al. Mutation of the human circadian clock gene CRY1 in familial delayed sleep phase disorder. Cell 2017;169(2):203–15.e13.
6. Trotti LM. Idiopathic hypersomnia. Sleep Med Clin 2017;12(3):331–44.
7. Sullivan SS, Kushida CA. Multiple sleep latency test and maintenance of wakefulness test. Chest 2008;134(4):854–61.
8. Huang YS, Guilleminault C, Lin CH, et al. Multiple sleep latency test in narcolepsy type 1 and narcolepsy type 2: a 5-year follow-up study. J Sleep Res 2018;27(5): e12700.
9. Trotti LM, Staab BA, Rye DB. Test-retest reliability of the multiple sleep latency test in narcolepsy without cataplexy and idiopathic hypersomnia. J Clin Sleep Med 2013;9(8):789–95.
10. Lopez R, Doukkali A, Barateau L, et al. Test-retest reliability of the multiple sleep latency test in central disorders of hypersomnolence. Sleep 2017;40(12):1–9.

11. Materna L, Halfter H, Heidbreder A, et al. Idiopathic hypersomnia patients revealed longer circadian period length in peripheral skin fibroblasts. Front Neurol 2018;9:424.

12. Lippert J, Halfter H, Heidbreder A, et al. Altered dynamics in the circadian oscillation of clock genes in dermal fibroblasts of patients suffering from idiopathic hypersomnia. PLoS One 2014;9(1):e85255.

13. Nevsimalova S, Blazejova K, Illnerova H, et al. A contribution to pathophysiology of idiopathic hypersomnia. Suppl Clin Neurophysiol 2000;53:366–70.

14. Pattyn N, Van Puyvelde M, Fernandez-Tellez H, et al. From the midnight sun to the longest night: Sleep in Antarctica. Sleep Med Rev 2018;37:159–72.

15. Paakkonen T, Leppaluoto J, Makinen TM, et al. Seasonal levels of melatonin, thyroid hormones, mood, and cognition near the Arctic Circle. Aviat Space Environ Med 2008;79(7):695–9.

16. Wehr TA, Duncan WC Jr, Sher L, et al. A circadian signal of change of season in patients with seasonal affective disorder. Arch Gen Psychiatry 2001;58(12):1108–14.

17. Aubin S, Kupers R, Ptito M, et al. Melatonin and cortisol profiles in the absence of light perception. Behav Brain Res 2017;317:515–21.

18. Stothard ER, McHill AW, Depner CM, et al. Circadian entrainment to the natural light-dark cycle across seasons and the weekend. Curr Biol 2017;27(4):508–13.

19. Aeschbach D, Sher L, Postolache TT, et al. A longer biological night in long sleepers than in short sleepers. J Clin Endocrinol Metab 2003;88(1):26–30.

20. Lane JM, Chang AM, Bjonnes AC, et al. Impact of common diabetes risk variant in MTNR1B on sleep, circadian, and melatonin physiology. Diabetes 2016;65(6):1741–51.

21. Ruoff C, Pizza F, Trotti LM, et al. The MSLT is repeatable in narcolepsy type 1 but not narcolepsy type 2: a retrospective patient study. J Clin Sleep Med 2018;14(1):65–74.

22. Ali M, Auger RR, Slocumb NL, et al. Idiopathic hypersomnia: clinical features and response to treatment. J Clin Sleep Med 2009;5(6):562–8.

23. Thakrar C, Patel K, D'Ancona G, et al. Effectiveness and side-effect profile of stimulant therapy as monotherapy and in combination in the central hypersomnias in clinical practice. J Sleep Res 2018;27(4):e12627.

24. Rosenthal NE, Jacobsen FM, Sack DA, et al. Atenolol in seasonal affective disorder: a test of the melatonin hypothesis. Am J Psychiatry 1988;145(1):52–6.

25. Schlager DS. Early-morning administration of short-acting beta blockers for treatment of winter depression. Am J Psychiatry 1994;151(9):1383–5.

26. Leu-Semenescu S, Louis P, Arnulf I. Benefits and risk of sodium oxybate in idiopathic hypersomnia versus narcolepsy type 1: a chart review. Sleep Med 2016;17:38–44.

27. Brismar K, Hylander B, Eliasson K, et al. Melatonin secretion related to side-effects of beta-blockers from the central nervous system. Acta Med Scand 1988;223(6):525–30.

28. Fares A. Night-time exogenous melatonin administration may be a beneficial treatment for sleeping disorders in beta blocker patients. J Cardiovasc Dis Res 2011;2(3):153–5.

29. Carpizo R, Martinez A, Mediavilla D, et al. Smith-Magenis syndrome: a case report of improved sleep after treatment with beta1-adrenergic antagonists and melatonin. J Pediatr 2006;149(3):409–11.

30. De Leersnyder H, Bresson JL, de Blois MC, et al. Beta 1-adrenergic antagonists and melatonin reset the clock and restore sleep in a circadian disorder, Smith-Magenis syndrome. J Med Genet 2003;40(1):74–8.

31. Auger RR, Burgess HJ, Emens JS, et al. Clinical practice guideline for the treatment of intrinsic circadian rhythm sleep-wake disorders: advanced sleep-wake phase disorder (ASWPD), delayed sleep-wake phase disorder (DSWPD), non-24-hour sleep-wake rhythm disorder (N24SWD), and irregular sleep-wake rhythm disorder (ISWRD). An update for 2015: an American Academy of Sleep Medicine Clinical Practice Guideline. J Clin Sleep Med 2015;11(10):1199–236.

32. Bruyneel M, Serste T. Sleep disturbances in patients with liver cirrhosis: prevalence, impact, and management challenges. Nat Sci Sleep 2018;10:369–75.

33. Formentin C, Garrido M, Montagnese S. Assessment and management of sleep disturbance in cirrhosis. Curr Hepatol Rep 2018;17(1):52–69.

34. Saleh K, Javaheri S. Sleep in ambulatory patients with stable cirrhosis of the liver. Sleep Med 2018;41:15–9.

35. Coy DL, Mehta R, Zee P, et al. Portal-systemic shunting and the disruption of circadian locomotor activity in the rat. Gastroenterology 1992;103(1):222–8.

36. Zee PC, Mehta R, Turek FW, et al. Portacaval anastomosis disrupts circadian locomotor activity and pineal melatonin rhythms in rats. Brain Res 1991;560(1–2):17–22.

37. Steindl PE, Ferenci P, Marktl W. Impaired hepatic catabolism of melatonin in cirrhosis. Ann Intern Med 1997;127(6):494.

38. Steindl PE, Finn B, Bendok B, et al. Disruption of the diurnal rhythm of plasma melatonin in cirrhosis. Ann Intern Med 1995;123(4):274–7.

39. Celinski K, Konturek PC, Slomka M, et al. Altered basal and postprandial plasma melatonin, gastrin, ghrelin, leptin and insulin in patients with liver cirrhosis and portal hypertension without and with oral administration of melatonin or tryptophan. J Pineal Res 2009;46(4):408–14.

40. Borodkin K, Ayalon L, Kanety H, et al. Dysregulation of circadian rhythms following prolactin-secreting pituitary microadenoma. Chronobiol Int 2005;22(1):145–56.

41. Schwartz WJ, Busis NA, Hedley-Whyte ET. A discrete lesion of ventral hypothalamus and optic chiasm that disturbed the daily temperature rhythm. J Neurol 1986;233(1):1–4.

42. Pardasani V, Shukla G, Singh S, et al. Abnormal sleep-wake cycles in patients with tuberculous meningitis: a case-control study. J Neurol Sci 2008;269(1–2):126–32.

43. Abreu T, Braganca M. The bipolarity of light and dark: a review on Bipolar Disorder and circadian cycles. J Affect Disord 2015;185:219–29.

44. Takaesu Y. Circadian rhythm in bipolar disorder: a review of the literature. Psychiatry Clin Neurosci 2018;72(9):673–82.

45. Melo MC, Garcia RF, Linhares Neto VB, et al. Sleep and circadian alterations in people at risk for bipolar disorder: a systematic review. J Psychiatr Res 2016;83:211–9.

46. McCarthy MJ, Welsh DK. Cellular circadian clocks in mood disorders. J Biol Rhythms 2012;27(5):339–52.

47. Iwahana E, Akiyama M, Miyakawa K, et al. Effect of lithium on the circadian rhythms of locomotor activity and glycogen synthase kinase-3 protein expression in the mouse suprachiasmatic nuclei. Eur J Neurosci 2004;19(8):2281–7.

48. Li J, Lu WQ, Beesley S, et al. Lithium impacts on the amplitude and period of the molecular circadian clockwork. PLoS One 2012;7(3):e33292.

49. Roybal K, Theobold D, Graham A, et al. Mania-like behavior induced by disruption of CLOCK. Proc Natl Acad Sci U S A 2007;104(15):6406–11.
50. Kristensen M, Nierenberg AA, Ostergaard SD. Face and predictive validity of the ClockDelta19 mouse as an animal model for bipolar disorder: a systematic review. Mol Psychiatry 2018;23(1):70–80.
51. Burgess HJ, Park M, Wyatt JK, et al. Sleep and circadian variability in people with delayed sleep-wake phase disorder versus healthy controls. Sleep Med 2017;34: 33–9.
52. Murray JM, Sletten TL, Magee M, et al. Prevalence of circadian misalignment and its association with depressive symptoms in delayed sleep phase disorder. Sleep 2017;40(1):1–10.
53. Liebzeit D, Phelan C, Moon C, et al. Rest-activity patterns in older adults with heart failure and healthy older adults. J Aging Phys Act 2017;25(1):116–22.
54. Jeon S, Conley S, Redeker NS. Discrepancy between wrist-actigraph and polysomnographic measures of sleep in patients with stable heart failure and a novel approach to evaluating discrepancy. J Sleep Res 2018;28:e12717.
55. Tan MKH, Wong JKL, Bakrania K, et al. Can activity monitors predict outcomes in patients with heart failure? A systematic review. Eur Heart J Qual Care Clin Outcomes 2019;5(1):11–21.
56. Chang AM, Aeschbach D, Duffy JF, et al. Evening use of light-emitting eReaders negatively affects sleep, circadian timing, and next-morning alertness. Proc Natl Acad Sci U S A 2015;112(4):1232–7.
57. Touitou Y, Touitou D, Reinberg A. Disruption of adolescents' circadian clock: the vicious circle of media use, exposure to light at night, sleep loss and risk behaviors. J Physiol Paris 2016;110(4 Pt B):467–79.
58. McHill AW, Phillips AJ, Czeisler CA, et al. Later circadian timing of food intake is associated with increased body fat. Am J Clin Nutr 2017;106(5):1213–9.
59. Morris CJ, Purvis TE, Mistretta J, et al. Circadian misalignment increases C-reactive protein and blood pressure in chronic shift workers. J Biol Rhythms 2017; 32(2):154–64.
60. Qian J, Dalla Man C, Morris CJ, et al. Differential effects of the circadian system and circadian misalignment on insulin sensitivity and insulin secretion in humans. Diabetes Obes Metab 2018;20(10):2481–5.
61. Qian J, Scheer F. Circadian system and glucose metabolism: implications for physiology and disease. Trends Endocrinol Metab 2016;27(5):282–93.
62. Stenvers DJ, Scheer F, Schrauwen P, et al. Circadian clocks and insulin resistance. Nat Rev Endocrinol 2019;15(2):75–89.
63. Vetter C, Dashti HS, Lane JM, et al. Night shift work, genetic risk, and type 2 diabetes in the UK biobank. Diabetes Care 2018;41(4):762–9.
64. Vetter C, Scheer F. Circadian biology: uncoupling human body clocks by food timing. Curr Biol 2017;27(13):R656–8.

Circadian Rhythms
Implications for Health and Disease

Sabra M. Abbott, MD, PhD[a], Phyllis C. Zee, MD, PhD[b],*

KEYWORDS

• Circadian • Aging • Cardiometabolic disease • Neurodegeneration

KEY POINTS

• Circadian rhythms are present throughout the body, and proper coordination of these rhythms is important for overall health.
• Circadian dysregulation has been associated with increased risk for cardiometabolic, neurologic, and neurodegenerative disease.
• Further studies are needed on the efficacy of targeted circadian-based interventions for improving cardiometabolic and neurologic health.

INTRODUCTION

Innate circadian (approximately a day) rhythms are ubiquitous in nearly all organisms, from single cells to humans. In just the past 50 years, it has become evident that these endogenous near 24-hour rhythms regulate not only the timing, but also the function of thousands of physiologic processes at the molecular, cellular, tissue, and organ levels.[1,2] In the 1980s, the discovery of circadian clock genes in flies[3–6] and nearly a decade later mammalian clock genes,[7] led to major breakthroughs in our understanding of the core molecular circadian clock machinery. The discovery that circadian clocks are found in nearly all cells and tissues, and among other functions, regulate cellular bioenergetics, inflammation, and cell division, has broadened our view of the importance of biological timing in health and disease. Indeed, there is mounting evidence that disruption of circadian clock function results in physiologic and behavioral aberrations, alterations, and dysfunctions that are relevant for the development of disease.[8] Circadian misalignment is associated with, and possibly contributes to, numerous diseases and disorders affecting nearly all systems of the body, including those related to neurologic, immune, and cardiometabolic function.[9]

Disclosure Statement: This article was in part supported by Northwestern University Feinberg School of Medicine Center for Circadian and Sleep Medicine.
[a] Department of Neurology, Northwestern University Feinberg School of Medicine, 710 North Lake Shore Drive, Abbott Hall 524, Chicago, IL 60611, USA; [b] Department of Neurology, Northwestern University Feinberg School of Medicine, 710 North Lake Shore Drive, Abbott Hall 521, Chicago, IL 60611, USA
* Corresponding author.
E-mail address: p-zee@northwestern.edu

In the past 150 years, with the advent and widespread use of electrical lighting, and more recently, the use of technology and personal light-emitting devices, humans have had the opportunity to override the inherent relationships among sleep, feeding, and activity with the natural physical cycles of light and darkness. Moreover, advances in technology and social media have facilitated the globalization of a 24/7 society, which further disrupts circadian physiology by misaligning sleep-wake behavior, and endogenous circadian rhythms with not only the natural light-dark cycle, but also among internal clocks in different tissues and organs. In humans, proper circadian organization (circadian health) is being increasingly threatened in our society by unhealthy lifestyle and chronic diseases, leading to circadian misalignment and sleep deficiency, which together can lead to adverse health outcomes. Disruption of internal temporal organization causes physiologic dysfunction and promotes susceptibility to numerous mental and physical diseases,[10–13] but in turn, medical diseases, such as many neurologic disorders, can contribute to circadian and sleep disturbances.[14] This article reviews the recent advances in the role of circadian clocks in aging and the expression and development of common cardiometabolic and neurologic disorders, along with general approaches to enhance the concept of circadian health.

AGING

The rapid global growth of our aging population, and associated age-related increase in chronic mental and medical disorders, are significant challenges for our society. The sleep-circadian health relationship is particularly significant because of increase in sleep and circadian disturbances in older adults, and the recognition of their contribution to cardiometabolic disorders and neurologic disease. Decreased circadian amplitude, increased instability, and internal desynchronization of physiologic and behavioral rhythms, such as sleep-wake rhythms, are common features of aging in humans and other mammals.[15,16] Furthermore, similar changes in circadian amplitude have been shown in neurochemical and neuroanatomical outputs of the suprachiasmatic nucleus (SCN)[17] and in the ability of the SCN to harmonize the symphony of rhythmic functions throughout the brain and body. Although the mechanisms of how these age-related changes result in neurodegenerative and cardiometabolic disorders are not fully understood, postulated pathways include alterations in key metabolic, immune, and inflammatory functions. In addition, weakening of environmental and social circadian synchronizing agents, such as decreased light exposure, the absence of work and activity schedules, or common age-related loss of photoreception, can negatively affect circadian function.[18–20] Interestingly, cataract surgery can have a positive effect on sleep quality.[21] **Fig. 1** provides a summary of the multiple extrinsic and intrinsic factors that can contribute to circadian disruption, as well as the proposed mechanisms linking circadian function and health.

The classic thinking was that these changes were a consequence of aging or age-related disease, and thus treatment was aimed at managing the associated sleep-wake disturbance. In the past decade, however, mounting data from animal and human studies indicate that impaired coordination in the timing and function between the SCN and clocks in various other brain and peripheral tissues may contribute to neurologic and metabolic aging.[22] Indeed, recent findings support the hypothesis that strengthening the circadian system may be a novel strategy to optimize the aging trajectory and reduce risk for neurodegeneration and cardiometabolic disease (CMD).[23–25]

CARDIOMETABOLIC DISEASE

CMD and the associated medical, neurologic, and psychiatric comorbidities remain some of the greatest public health challenges of the twenty-first century. Although

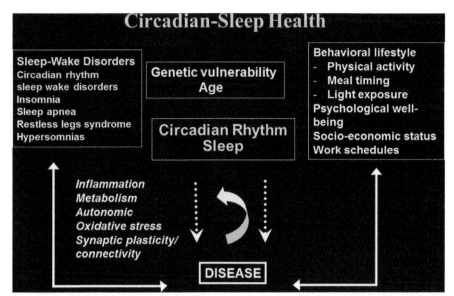

Fig. 1. Outline of potential factors mediating the interaction between sleep/circadian dysfunction and neurodegenerative disease risk.

circadian rhythm alterations have been linked to multiple medical and psychiatric disease states, including immunologic, neoplastic, and mood disorders, it can be argued that the most advanced area for understanding the importance and the underlying pathways have come from studies of body weight regulation and metabolic function.[26] There has been increasing recognition that disrupted circadian function represents a significant risk factor for CMD, and that these adverse effects may be even more pronounced in patients with CMD. It is important to note that cardiovascular and metabolic health has implications for the function of a broad range of tissues and organs, including the nervous system.

The discovery that the *Clock* mutant mouse becomes obese opened up new avenues of research on how metabolic and circadian clock genes interact with one another and how long-term circadian disruption impacts cardiometabolic health.[27] The finding that behavioral, as well as peripheral and central molecular clock rhythms were altered in mice fed a high-fat diet[28] led to new insights into how metabolic gene loops are interlocked with core circadian clock gene loops and in turn can alter circadian timing and potentially also sleep. The finding that mice who are allowed to eat only during the "wrong" time of day gain more weight than mice fed at the "right" time of day[29,30] has led to the recognition of the importance of the circadian clock and the time of food intake on the epidemic of obesity, diabetes, and cardiovascular disease in many modern societies.

In humans, evidence points to a relationship between late bedtimes and meals with higher caloric intake, increased consumption of unhealthy foods,[31] and higher body mass index.[32,33] Consistent with these observations is the emerging data showing that a later or evening circadian chronotype is associated with higher HbA1c in patients with diabetes.[34] One of the most common causes of chronic circadian misalignment in our society is shift work. There is ample evidence that shift work increases the risk for cardiometabolic disorders, including diabetes, heart disease, hypertension, and cognitive impairment.[35–39] There is also evidence that experimentally induced circadian misalignment increases measures of CMD risk in both animals and humans.[12,13,30] Together, these findings, support a bidirectional relationship between circadian disruption and CMD. However, there are major remaining questions regarding the mechanisms of this clock-CMD relationship, and how the coordination between central and peripheral clocks affect metabolic processes.

Circadian-based approaches have been investigated as potential novel treatments for CMD and associated comorbidities, including cancer. In addition to timed exposure to bright light[40] and physical activity,[41] meal timing can serve as an important metabolic clock signal. The benefits of time-restricted feeding on metabolic[30] and cardiovascular[42] measures have been demonstrated in animals. An emerging limited number of studies in humans also show that restricting feeding to a specified 10-hour to 12-hour window during the day can have positive effects on body weight and sleep quality.[30,42]

NEUROLOGIC DISEASE

Circadian rhythms in behavioral, hormonal, and physiologic rhythms, including the 24-hour sleep-wake cycle are often disrupted in patients with neurologic disorders.[43] It was commonly assumed that the circadian disturbance, which is mainly clinically manifested by changes in sleep and wakefulness, was secondary to the underlying neurologic disorder, and treatments were aimed at symptomatic management. In the past decade, the fundamental discovery of the role of circadian clock genes in the regulation of neuronal function,[44] and that disruption of clock function can alter the expression and development of neurologic disorders, supports the view that circadian dysfunction may play a role in the pathophysiology of some neuronal disorders, or could be manipulated to improve treatment outcomes. Although circadian rhythms likely play a role in many neurologic conditions, such as stroke, multiple sclerosis, and neuromuscular disorders, in this section, we discuss a few examples of some common neurologic disorders in which circadian rhythm disturbances have been well described, including epilepsy, headache, and neurodegenerative disorders.

Epilepsy

It is well known that there are temporal patterns in seizure frequency, particularly the day-night or sleep-wake occurrence, and that sleep and arousal states influence the expression of seizure activity.[45,46] The relationship between circadian chronotype and epilepsy types have yielded conflicting results.[47–49] Most of the studies in this area were descriptive, but technological advances in long-term electroencephalogram monitoring and analytical tools have provided new insights into the role of circadian rhythms in the regulation of neuronal excitatory and inhibitory activity, and vulnerability to seizure propagation.[47] Interestingly, although interictal epileptiform activity is higher in sleep, ictal state appears to be modulated by circadian rhythmicity.[50] Circadian rhythms can affect seizure timing, frequency, and even severity by the rhythmic regulation of neuronal activity, and the regulation of sleep and wake timing. For example, cortical excitability has been shown to be lower in the evening than during the day[51] and increases with time awake.[52,53]

The interaction between circadian-regulated cortical excitability and sleep state may explain the clinical observation of increased seizure activity with sleep deprivation. At the molecular level, the core circadian clock genes, *BMAL1* and *CLOCK*, have been shown to regulate neuronal excitability and thus ictal threshold.[54–57] The evidence strongly supports an interaction between vigilance and sleep states on seizures. However, the relative influence of sleep-arousal states or circadian modulation on seizure expression may depend on seizure type, age, and other environmental and behavioral variables. Nevertheless, consideration of circadian influences may predict seizure timing and the optimal timing of tailored medication regimens in patients. Assessing circadian chronotype also may be useful in aligning circadian timing with sleep-wake activity, as well as timing of medications to optimize seizure control.

Headache

The most common types of headaches that exhibit a circadian pattern and are influenced by sleep or vigilance states are migraine, cluster, and paroxysmal hemicranias.[58] The interactions between sleep and circadian modulation of vascular function, neurotransmitter (histamine, serotonin) levels, and pain threshold are likely involved in the temporal distribution of the frequency and perhaps also severity of these headaches.

In this section, we focus the discussion on migraine, the most common of these types.[59] It has been well recognized that sleep disturbances are common and contribute to the development of chronic migraine.[60,61] Although circadian rhythms are essential in the regulation of the timing and quality of sleep, studies on the role of circadian factors in migraine have been limited and largely descriptive. There is a suggestion that patients with migraine exhibit a delay in the timing of circadian rhythms, as measured by dim-light melatonin onset (DLMO), and a lower amplitude of the melatonin rhythm.[62-65] These findings led to several small treatment trials with exogenous melatonin, indicating a potential beneficial effect on acute and subacute migraine control.[66-68]

The emerging evidence of the detrimental effects of circadian misalignment on disease risk, and technological advances in the measurement of circadian biomarkers, such as melatonin, have resulted in a resurgence of interest on the relationship between circadian misalignment and migraine. A recent study of 2875 patients with migraine and 200 controls, evaluated the correlation between circadian chronotype self-reported circadian stability (using Circadian Type Inventory) with the timing of migraine events.[69] The results found that patients with migraine were more likely to be early chronotypes or delayed chronotypes compared with controls, and more migraine events occurred in the morning. Another study went a step further to determine whether circadian misalignment exacerbated migraines.[70] This pilot study assessed circadian rhythm and phase by DLMO and actigraphy in 20 patients and 20 controls. Within the migraine group, a higher frequency of attacks was correlated with a later circadian phase, and a larger phase angle between DLMO and sleep timing was correlated with higher migraine-related disability.

Although the evidence is limited, the results support a role for circadian dysfunction in migraine, with circadian misalignment exacerbating migraines. The finding of a common gene mutation in familial migraine and familial advanced sleep-wake phase disorder provides further support for circadian involvement in the expression of migraine. Circadian-based approaches, such as timed light, melatonin, and physical activity, to improve circadian alignment between endogenous circadian rhythm and sleep and other behaviors have the potential to improve the management of headaches, such as migraine, but also other headache types.

Neurodegenerative Disease

Circadian rhythm and sleep disturbances are highly prevalent in neurodegenerative disorders such as Alzheimer disease (AD), Parkinson disease (PD), Huntington disease, and traumatic brain injury. Characteristic findings in most of these conditions are a decrease in the amplitude or day-night robustness or a change (typically delay) in the phase of the circadian rhythm of sleep-wake and other physiologic rhythms with respect to the environment.[71-79] Emerging new evidence indicates that not only are sleep and circadian disturbances common, but they likely also contribute to the expression and development of neurodegeneration.[75] Although the pathways linking circadian rhythms and neuronal health are likely multifactorial, including alterations in metabolism, oxidative stress, and inflammation, recent evidence points to neuroinflammation as a potential common pathway.[80] The investigators demonstrate that the circadian clock component, Rev-erbα is a mediator of microglial activation and neuroinflammation in the hippocampus of mice. These results suggest that circadian dysregulation alters inflammatory processes, which in turn can affect neuronal health. In this section, we focus the discussion on the 2 most common neurodegenerative disorders: AD and PD.

Alzheimer disease and other dementias

Sleep-wake fragmentation is a characteristic feature of AD, affecting nearly 40% of patients with dementia,[81,82] with even higher rates in the late stages of the disease. This type of sleep-wake pattern is consistent with irregular sleep-wake rhythm disorder (ISWRD). The fragmentation of nocturnal sleep and daytime alertness negatively affects the quality of life of the patient and the caregiver. In addition to the underlying disease, behavioral and environmental factors, such as decreased light exposure,[83] lack of structured social and physical activities,[84] side effects of medications, and other sleep disorders such as sleep apnea, can contribute to sleep and wake disturbances. Investigators have used timed exposure to bright light[85–88]; structured activities[89,90]; pharmacotherapy with hypnotic, antipsychotic, antidepressant medications[91]; and melatonin (sometimes in high doses) to help consolidate sleep and enhance daytime wakefulness. In general, a combination of increased light exposure during the day and daytime structuring of activities can be beneficial.[92,93] Supplementation with melatonin at night has had mixed results.[94] More detailed treatment approaches for ISWRD associated with dementia are discussed in Temitayo Oyegbile and Aleksandar Videnovic's article, "Irregular Sleep Wake Rhythm Sleep-Wake Disorders," elsewhere in this issue.

The concept that circadian and sleep disturbances represent early risk factors for AD has gained momentum, both in terms of research, as well as recognition by the neurologic community. There is a growing body of evidence from epidemiologic studies that fragmentation of the circadian sleep-wake rhythm precedes clinical cognitive impairment by several decades,[95,96] and its potential as an early biomarker of neurodegeneration. Because circadian rhythms regulate sleep-wake function, it is in practice difficult to separate the circadian and sleep contributions to AD pathophysiology. For example, dysfunction of circadian regulation will affect the ability to consolidate sleep, and in turn may affect the amount of slow wave sleep, which has been found to be important for cognitive health.[97] Specifically, sleep disturbance and impairment in slow wave sleep have been shown to increase neuronal excitability and decreased clearance of Aβ levels in the cerebrospinal fluid.[98–100]

Interventions aimed at strengthening the amplitude and stability of circadian rhythms using behavioral and environmental therapies have shown promise in improving sleep-wake disturbance and reducing cognitive deterioration in patients with dementia. However, definitive trials using either behavioral or pharmacologic therapies are generally lacking. Improved understanding of the molecular, cellular, physiologic, and behavioral mechanisms linking circadian rhythms with neuronal health and neural networks involved in cognition can offer opportunities for the development of circadian-based diagnostics and therapies for AD and related dementias.

Parkinson disease

Sleep problems are common in patients with PD. Along with the more commonly described problems of rapid-eye movement behavior disorder, insomnia, and daytime sleepiness, these patients often exhibit circadian rhythm abnormalities. Similar to the patterns seen in AD, the circadian disruption is believed to be both a reflection of underlying neurodegeneration, as well as a potential inciting factor for further disease progression. The most frequent pattern of circadian disruption observed in PD is a decrease in circadian amplitude, which can be measured in daily rest-activity patterns,[101] levels of melatonin and cortisol,[102–104] and daily blood pressure rhythms.[105]

Multiple factors associated with PD may contribute to the observed circadian dysfunction. At the level of input to the circadian clock, dopamine levels in the retina can influence the expression of melanopsin in retinal ganglion cells, which provide light input to the SCN.[106] Loss of dopamine with PD can then in turn influence the ability of environmental light information to reach the central circadian pacemaker. There is also evidence of neurodegeneration directly at the level of the SCN.[107] Degeneration at the level of the SCN can in turn can affect circadian outputs, such as the pattern and amplitude of melatonin release. Along with serving as a marker of circadian timing, melatonin also plays multiple other roles throughout the body. Most importantly for patients with PD, it acts to inhibit the expression of α-synuclein.[108,109] Abnormal accumulation of α-synuclein is thought to play a major role in the underlying pathogenesis of PD. In addition, similar to AD, there is growing evidence that the circadian disruption associated with PD can in turn increase the risk for further disease progression.[110]

There are exciting advances looking at the ability of circadian-based interventions to improve clinical outcomes in patients with PD. Melatonin administered at bedtime has been demonstrated to improve sleep quality and daytime sleepiness.[85,111] More recently, several studies have looked at the use of bright-light therapy in the morning,[112] before bedtime,[113] or twice daily,[114] and in all cases patients have demonstrated an improvement in sleep. Overall, this remains a promising area for future research into sleep/circadian-based interventions to improve symptoms and even potentially slow disease progression.

SUMMARY

Overall, there is growing evidence that proper alignment between the circadian clock and external environment, and between circadian processes within an individual, are important for overall health. Circadian dysregulation can be both a marker and a perpetuator of disease processes. With this growing knowledge comes the opportunity to provide novel interventions to strengthen circadian rhythms, with a goal of improving overall health.

REFERENCES

1. Stephan FK, Zucker I. Circadian rhythms in drinking behavior and locomotor activity of rats are eliminated by hypothalamic lesions. Proc Natl Acad Sci U S A 1972;69(6):1583–6.
2. Mohawk JA, Green CB, Takahashi JS. Central and peripheral circadian clocks in mammals. Annu Rev Neurosci 2012;35:445–62.
3. Reddy P, Zehring WA, Wheeler DA, et al. Molecular analysis of the period locus in *Drosophila melanogaster* and identification of a transcript involved in biological rhythms. Cell 1984;38(3):701–10.
4. Zehring WA, Wheeler DA, Reddy P, et al. P-element transformation with period locus DNA restores rhythmicity to mutant, arrhythmic *Drosophila melanogaster*. Cell 1984;39(2 Pt 1):369–76.

5. Bargiello TA, Young MW. Molecular genetics of a biological clock in *Drosophila*. Proc Natl Acad Sci U S A 1984;81(7):2142–6.
6. Jackson FR, Bargiello TA, Yun SH, et al. Product of per locus of Drosophila shares homology with proteoglycans. Nature 1986;320(6058):185–8.
7. Vitaterna MH, King DP, Chang AM, et al. Mutagenesis and mapping of a mouse gene, *Clock*, essential for circadian behavior. Science 1994;264(5159):719–25.
8. Jagannath A, Taylor L, Wakaf Z, et al. The genetics of circadian rhythms, sleep and health. Hum Mol Genet 2017;26(R2):R128–38.
9. Summa KC, Turek FW. Chronobiology and obesity: interactions between circadian rhythms and energy regulation. Adv Nutr 2014;5(3):312S–9S.
10. Hardeland R, Madrid JA, Tan DX, et al. Melatonin, the circadian multioscillator system and health: the need for detailed analyses of peripheral melatonin signaling. J Pineal Res 2012;52(2):139–66.
11. Zee PC, Turek FW. Respect the clock. Sleep Med Rev 2013;17(6):395–7.
12. Scheer FA, Hilton MF, Mantzoros CS, et al. Adverse metabolic and cardiovascular consequences of circadian misalignment. Proc Natl Acad Sci U S A 2009; 106(11):4453–8.
13. McHill AW, Melanson EL, Higgins J, et al. Impact of circadian misalignment on energy metabolism during simulated nightshift work. Proc Natl Acad Sci U S A 2014;111(48):17302–7.
14. Ju YS, Videnovic A, Vaughn BV. Comorbid sleep disturbances in neurologic disorders. Continuum (Minneap Minn) 2017;23(4):1117–31.
15. Youngstedt SD, Kripke DF, Elliott JA, et al. Circadian abnormalities in older adults. J Pineal Res 2001;31(3):264–72.
16. Hofman MA. The human circadian clock and aging. Chronobiol Int 2000;17(3):245–59.
17. Nakamura TJ, Nakamura W, Yamazaki S, et al. Age-related decline in circadian output. J Neurosci 2011;31(28):10201–5.
18. Obayashi K, Saeki K, Tone N, et al. Lower melatonin secretion in older females: gender differences independent of light exposure profiles. J Epidemiol 2015; 25(1):38–43.
19. Banks G, Heise I, Starbuck B, et al. Genetic background influences age-related decline in visual and nonvisual retinal responses, circadian rhythms, and sleep. Neurobiol Aging 2015;36(1):380–93.
20. Munch M, Schmieder M, Bieler K, et al. Bright light delights: effects of daily light exposure on emotions, rest-activity cycles, sleep and melatonin secretion in severely demented patients. Curr Alzheimer Res 2017;14(10):1063–75.
21. Alexander I, Cuthbertson FM, Ratnarajan G, et al. Impact of cataract surgery on sleep in patients receiving either ultraviolet-blocking or blue-filtering intraocular lens implants. Invest Ophthalmol Vis Sci 2014;55(8):4999–5004.
22. Musiek ES, Bhimasani M, Zangrilli MA, et al. Circadian rest-activity pattern changes in aging and preclinical Alzheimer disease. JAMA Neurol 2018; 75(5):582–90.
23. Whittaker DS, Loh DH, Wang HB, et al. Circadian-based treatment strategy effective in the BACHD mouse model of Huntington's disease. J Biol Rhythms 2018;33(5):535–54.
24. Takahashi M, Haraguchi A, Tahara Y, et al. Positive association between physical activity and PER3 expression in older adults. Sci Rep 2017;7:39771.
25. Wang HB, Loh DH, Whittaker DS, et al. Time-restricted feeding improves circadian dysfunction as well as motor symptoms in the Q175 mouse model of Huntington's disease. eNeuro 2018;5(1) [pii:ENEURO.0431-17.2017].

26. Summa K, Turek F. The clocks within us. Sci Am 2015;312(2):50–5.
27. Turek FW, Joshu C, Kohsaka A, et al. Obesity and metabolic syndrome in circadian Clock mutant mice. Science 2005;308(5724):1043–5.
28. Kohsaka A, Laposky AD, Ramsey KM, et al. High-fat diet disrupts behavioral and molecular circadian rhythms in mice. Cell Metab 2007;6(5):414–21.
29. Arble DM, Bass J, Laposky AD, et al. Circadian timing of food intake contributes to weight gain. Obesity (Silver Spring) 2009;17(11):2100–2.
30. Hatori M, Vollmers C, Zarrinpar A, et al. Time-restricted feeding without reducing caloric intake prevents metabolic diseases in mice fed a high-fat diet. Cell Metab 2012;15(6):848–60.
31. Reid KJ, Baron KG, Zee PC. Meal timing influences daily caloric intake in healthy adults. Nutr Res 2014;34(11):930–5.
32. Baron KG, Reid KJ, Kern AS, et al. Role of sleep timing in caloric intake and BMI. Obesity (Silver Spring) 2011;19(7):1374–81.
33. Reid KJ, Santostasi G, Baron KG, et al. Timing and intensity of light correlate with body weight in adults. PLoS One 2014;9(4):e92251.
34. Reutrakul S, Hood MM, Crowley SJ, et al. Chronotype is independently associated with glycemic control in type 2 diabetes. Diabetes Care 2013;36(9):2523–9.
35. Spiegel K, Leproult R, Van Cauter E. Impact of sleep debt on metabolic and endocrine function. Lancet 1999;354(9188):1435–9.
36. Knutsson A, Kempe A. Shift work and diabetes–a systematic review. Chronobiol Int 2014;31(10):1146–51.
37. Manohar S, Thongprayoon C, Cheungpasitporn W, et al. Associations of rotational shift work and night shift status with hypertension: a systematic review and meta-analysis. J Hypertens 2017;35(10):1929–37.
38. Vetter C, Devore EE, Wegrzyn LR, et al. Association between rotating night shift work and risk of coronary heart disease among women. JAMA 2016;315(16):1726–34.
39. Kecklund G, Axelsson J. Health consequences of shift work and insufficient sleep. BMJ 2016;355:i5210.
40. Khalsa SB, Jewett ME, Cajochen C, et al. A phase response curve to single bright light pulses in human subjects. J Physiol 2003;549(Pt 3):945–52.
41. Buxton OM, Lee CW, L'Hermite-Baleriaux M, et al. Exercise elicits phase shifts and acute alterations of melatonin that vary with circadian phase. Am J Physiol Regul Integr Comp Physiol 2003;284(3):R714–24.
42. Gill S, Le HD, Melkani GC, et al. Time-restricted feeding attenuates age-related cardiac decline in *Drosophila*. Science 2015;347(6227):1265–9.
43. Turek FW, Dugovic C, Zee PC. Current understanding of the circadian clock and the clinical implications for neurological disorders. Arch Neurol 2001;58(11):1781–7.
44. Leng Y, Musiek ES, Hu K, et al. Association between circadian rhythms and neurodegenerative diseases. Lancet Neurol 2019;18(3):307–18.
45. Crespel A, Coubes P, Baldy-Moulinier M. Sleep influence on seizures and epilepsy effects on sleep in partial frontal and temporal lobe epilepsies. Clin Neurophysiol 2000;111(Suppl 2):S54–9.
46. Malow BA. Sleep and epilepsy. Neurol Clin 1996;14(4):765–89.
47. Khan S, Nobili L, Khatami R, et al. Circadian rhythm and epilepsy. Lancet Neurol 2018;17(12):1098–108.
48. Kendis H, Baron K, Schuele SU, et al. Chronotypes in patients with epilepsy: does the type of epilepsy make a difference? Behav Neurol 2015;2015:941354.

49. Choi SJ, Joo EY, Hong SB. Sleep-wake pattern, chronotype and seizures in patients with epilepsy. Epilepsy Res 2016;120:19–24.

50. Spencer DC, Sun FT, Brown SN, et al. Circadian and ultradian patterns of epileptiform discharges differ by seizure-onset location during long-term ambulatory intracranial monitoring. Epilepsia 2016;57(9):1495–502.

51. Ly JQM, Gaggioni G, Chellappa SL, et al. Circadian regulation of human cortical excitability. Nat Commun 2016;7:11828.

52. Badawy RA, Curatolo JM, Newton M, et al. Sleep deprivation increases cortical excitability in epilepsy: syndrome-specific effects. Neurology 2006;67(6): 1018–22.

53. Muto V, Jaspar M, Meyer C, et al. Local modulation of human brain responses by circadian rhythmicity and sleep debt. Science 2016;353(6300):687–90.

54. Gerstner JR, Smith GG, Lenz O, et al. BMAL1 controls the diurnal rhythm and set point for electrical seizure threshold in mice. Front Syst Neurosci 2014;8:121.

55. Li P, Fu X, Smith NA, et al. Loss of CLOCK results in dysfunction of brain circuits underlying focal epilepsy. Neuron 2017;96(2):387–401 e6.

56. Scheffer IE, Heron SE, Regan BM, et al. Mutations in mammalian target of rapamycin regulator DEPDC5 cause focal epilepsy with brain malformations. Ann Neurol 2014;75(5):782–7.

57. Lipton JO, Yuan ED, Boyle LM, et al. The Circadian protein BMAL1 regulates translation in response to S6K1-mediated phosphorylation. Cell 2015;161(5): 1138–51.

58. Rovers J, Smits M, Duffy JF. Headache and sleep: also assess circadian rhythm sleep disorders. Headache 2014;54(1):175–7.

59. Paiva T, Farinha A, Martins A, et al. Chronic headaches and sleep disorders. Arch Intern Med 1997;157(15):1701–5.

60. Bigal ME, Lipton RB. Modifiable risk factors for migraine progression (or for chronic daily headaches)–clinical lessons. Headache 2006;46(Suppl 3):S144–6.

61. Kelman L, Rains JC. Headache and sleep: examination of sleep patterns and complaints in a large clinical sample of migraineurs. Headache 2005;45(7): 904–10.

62. Peres MF, Sanchez del Rio M, Seabra ML, et al. Hypothalamic involvement in chronic migraine. J Neurol Neurosurg Psychiatry 2001;71(6):747–51.

63. Claustrat B, Loisy C, Brun J, et al. Nocturnal plasma melatonin levels in migraine: a preliminary report. Headache 1989;29(4):242–5.

64. Brun J, Claustrat B, Saddier P, et al. Nocturnal melatonin excretion is decreased in patients with migraine without aura attacks associated with menses. Cephalalgia 1995;15(2):136–9 [discussion: 79].

65. Murialdo G, Fonzi S, Costelli P, et al. Urinary melatonin excretion throughout the ovarian cycle in menstrually related migraine. Cephalalgia 1994;14(3):205–9.

66. Claustrat B, Brun J, Geoffriau M, et al. Nocturnal plasma melatonin profile and melatonin kinetics during infusion in status migrainosus. Cephalalgia 1997; 17(4):511–7 [discussion: 487].

67. Nagtegaal JE, Smits MG, Swart AC, et al. Melatonin-responsive headache in delayed sleep phase syndrome: preliminary observations. Headache 1998;38(4): 303–7.

68. Goncalves AL, Martini Ferreira A, Ribeiro RT, et al. Randomised clinical trial comparing melatonin 3 mg, amitriptyline 25 mg and placebo for migraine prevention. J Neurol Neurosurg Psychiatry 2016;87(10):1127–32.

69. van Oosterhout W, van Someren E, Schoonman GG, et al. Chronotypes and circadian timing in migraine. Cephalalgia 2018;38(4):617–25.

70. Ong JC, Taylor HL, Park M, et al. Can circadian dysregulation exacerbate migraines? Headache 2018;58(7):1040–51.
71. Morton AJ, Wood NI, Hastings MH, et al. Disintegration of the sleep-wake cycle and circadian timing in Huntington's disease. J Neurosci 2005;25(1):157–63.
72. Pallier PN, Maywood ES, Zheng Z, et al. Pharmacological imposition of sleep slows cognitive decline and reverses dysregulation of circadian gene expression in a transgenic mouse model of Huntington's disease. J Neurosci 2007; 27(29):7869–78.
73. Skene DJ, Swaab DF. Melatonin rhythmicity: effect of age and Alzheimer's disease. Exp Gerontol 2003;38(1–2):199–206.
74. Witting W, Kwa IH, Eikelenboom P, et al. Alterations in the circadian rest-activity rhythm in aging and Alzheimer's disease. Biol Psychiatry 1990;27(6):563–72.
75. Musiek ES, Holtzman DM. Mechanisms linking circadian clocks, sleep, and neurodegeneration. Science 2016;354(6315):1004–8.
76. Schlosser Covell GE, Dhawan PS, Lee Iannotti JK, et al. Disrupted daytime activity and altered sleep-wake patterns may predict transition to mild cognitive impairment or dementia: a critically appraised topic. Neurologist 2012;18(6): 426–9.
77. Aziz NA, Pijl H, Frolich M, et al. Delayed onset of the diurnal melatonin rise in patients with Huntington's disease. J Neurol 2009;256(12):1961–5.
78. Boone DR, Sell SL, Micci MA, et al. Traumatic brain injury-induced dysregulation of the circadian clock. PLoS One 2012;7(10):e46204.
79. Mathias JL, Alvaro PK. Prevalence of sleep disturbances, disorders, and problems following traumatic brain injury: a meta-analysis. Sleep Med 2012;13(7): 898–905.
80. Griffin P, Dimitry JM, Sheehan PW, et al. Circadian clock protein Rev-erbalpha regulates neuroinflammation. Proc Natl Acad Sci U S A 2019;116(11):5102–7.
81. Ancoli-Israel S, Klauber MR, Butters N, et al. Dementia in institutionalized elderly: relation to sleep apnea. J Am Geriatr Soc 1991;39(3):258–63.
82. Zhao QF, Tan L, Wang HF, et al. The prevalence of neuropsychiatric symptoms in Alzheimer's disease: systematic review and meta-analysis. J Affect Disord 2016; 190:264–71.
83. Endo T, Kripke DF, Ancoli-Israel S. Wake up time, light, and mood in a population sample age 40-64 years. Psychiatry Investig 2015;12(2):177–82.
84. van Alphen HJ, Volkers KM, Blankevoort CG, et al. Older adults with dementia are sedentary for most of the day. PLoS One 2016;11(3):e0152457.
85. Dowling GA, Mastick J, Colling E, et al. Melatonin for sleep disturbances in Parkinson's disease. Sleep Med 2005;6(5):459–66.
86. Riemersma-van der Lek RF, Swaab DF, Twisk J, et al. Effect of bright light and melatonin on cognitive and noncognitive function in elderly residents of group care facilities: a randomized controlled trial. JAMA 2008;299(22):2642–55.
87. Ancoli-Israel S, Gehrman P, Martin JL, et al. Increased light exposure consolidates sleep and strengthens circadian rhythms in severe Alzheimer's disease patients. Behav Sleep Med 2003;1(1):22–36.
88. Sekiguchi H, Iritani S, Fujita K. Bright light therapy for sleep disturbance in dementia is most effective for mild to moderate Alzheimer's type dementia: a case series. Psychogeriatrics 2017;17(5):275–81.
89. Alessi CA, Schnelle JF, MacRae PG, et al. Does physical activity improve sleep in impaired nursing home residents? J Am Geriatr Soc 1995;43(10):1098–102.

90. Alessi CA, Yoon E, Schnelle JF, et al. A randomized trial of a combined physical activity and environmental intervention in nursing home residents: do sleep and agitation improve? J Am Geriatr Soc 1999;47(7):784–91.

91. Alessi CA, Schnelle JF, Traub S, et al. Psychotropic medications in incontinent nursing home residents: association with sleep and bed mobility. J Am Geriatr Soc 1995;43(7):788–92.

92. Alessi CA, Martin JL, Webber AP, et al. Randomized, controlled trial of a non-pharmacological intervention to improve abnormal sleep/wake patterns in nursing home residents. J Am Geriatr Soc 2005;53(5):803–10.

93. Martin JL, Marler MR, Harker JO, et al. A multicomponent nonpharmacological intervention improves activity rhythms among nursing home residents with disrupted sleep/wake patterns. J Gerontol A Biol Sci Med Sci 2007;62(1):67–72.

94. Wang YY, Zheng W, Ng CH, et al. Meta-analysis of randomized, double-blind, placebo-controlled trials of melatonin in Alzheimer's disease. Int J Geriatr Psychiatry 2017;32(1):50–7.

95. Lim AS, Kowgier M, Yu L, et al. Sleep fragmentation and the risk of incident Alzheimer's disease and cognitive decline in older persons. Sleep 2013;36(7):1027–32.

96. Shi L, Chen SJ, Ma MY, et al. Sleep disturbances increase the risk of dementia: a systematic review and meta-analysis. Sleep Med Rev 2018;40:4–16.

97. Tononi G, Cirelli C. Sleep and the price of plasticity: from synaptic and cellular homeostasis to memory consolidation and integration. Neuron 2014;81(1):12–34.

98. Xie L, Kang H, Xu Q, et al. Sleep drives metabolite clearance from the adult brain. Science 2013;342(6156):373–7.

99. Ooms S, Overeem S, Besse K, et al. Effect of 1 night of total sleep deprivation on cerebrospinal fluid beta-amyloid 42 in healthy middle-aged men: a randomized clinical trial. JAMA Neurol 2014;71(8):971–7.

100. Ju YS, Ooms SJ, Sutphen C, et al. Slow wave sleep disruption increases cerebrospinal fluid amyloid-beta levels. Brain 2017;140(8):2104–11.

101. van Hilten B, Hoff JI, Middelkoop HA, et al. Sleep disruption in Parkinson's disease. Assessment by continuous activity monitoring. Arch Neurol 1994;51(9):922–8.

102. Bordet R, Devos D, Brique S, et al. Study of circadian melatonin secretion pattern at different stages of Parkinson's disease. Clin Neuropharmacol 2003;26(2):65–72.

103. Fertl E, Auff E, Doppelbauer A, et al. Circadian secretion pattern of melatonin in de novo parkinsonian patients: evidence for phase-shifting properties of l-dopa. J Neural Transm Park Dis Dement Sect 1993;5(3):227–34.

104. Hartmann A, Veldhuis JD, Deuschle M, et al. Twenty-four hour cortisol release profiles in patients with Alzheimer's and Parkinson's disease compared to normal controls: ultradian secretory pulsatility and diurnal variation. Neurobiol Aging 1997;18(3):285–9.

105. Stuebner E, Vichayanrat E, Low DA, et al. Twenty-four hour non-invasive ambulatory blood pressure and heart rate monitoring in Parkinson's disease. Front Neurol 2013;4:49.

106. La Morgia C, Ross-Cisneros FN, Sadun AA, et al. Retinal ganglion cells and circadian rhythms in Alzheimer's Disease, Parkinson's Disease, and beyond. Front Neurol 2017;8:162.

107. De Pablo-Fernandez E, Courtney R, Warner TT, et al. A histologic study of the Circadian system in Parkinson disease, multiple system atrophy, and progressive supranuclear palsy. JAMA Neurol 2018;75(8):1008–12.
108. Sae-Ung K, Ueda K, Govitrapong P, et al. Melatonin reduces the expression of alpha-synuclein in the dopamine containing neuronal regions of amphetamine-treated postnatal rats. J Pineal Res 2012;52(1):128–37.
109. Ono K, Mochizuki H, Ikeda T, et al. Effect of melatonin on alpha-synuclein self-assembly and cytotoxicity. Neurobiol Aging 2012;33(9):2172–85.
110. Lauretti E, Di Meco A, Merali S, et al. Circadian rhythm dysfunction: a novel environmental risk factor for Parkinson's disease. Mol Psychiatry 2017;22(2):280–6.
111. Medeiros CA, Carvalhedo de Bruin PF, Lopes LA, et al. Effect of exogenous melatonin on sleep and motor dysfunction in Parkinson's disease. A randomized, double blind, placebo-controlled study. J Neurol 2007;254(4):459–64.
112. Paus S, Schmitz-Hubsch T, Wullner U, et al. Bright light therapy in Parkinson's disease: a pilot study. Mov Disord 2007;22(10):1495–8.
113. Willis GL, Moore C, Armstrong SM. A historical justification for and retrospective analysis of the systematic application of light therapy in Parkinson's disease. Rev Neurosci 2012;23(2):199–226.
114. Videnovic A, Klerman EB, Wang W, et al. Timed light therapy for sleep and daytime sleepiness associated with Parkinson disease: a randomized clinical trial. JAMA Neurol 2017;74(4):411–8.

Sleep and Circadian Medicine
Time of Day in the Neurologic Clinic

Marc D. Ruben, PhD[a,b,1], John B. Hogenesch, PhD[a,b,1],
David F. Smith, MD, PhD[c,d,e],*

KEYWORDS

- Circadian medicine • Chronotherapy • Sleep medicine • Neurology
- Circadian rhythms

KEY POINTS

- Fundamental neural processes are normally time-of-day regulated, likely explaining the tight link between disrupted circadian rhythms and neurologic disease.
- Time of day is rarely considered for central nervous system–targeting therapies. Circadian medicine incorporates knowledge of 24-hour biological rhythms to administer more effective treatment.
- It is conceivable that (1) determining a patient's internal circadian time, and (2) prescribing time-stipulated therapy will be common practice in neurology clinics in the coming decade.

INTRODUCTION
Rhythms in the Brain

Much of human biology is organized around the 24-hour day. Exercise, eating, digestion, and sleep occur at particular times, requiring highly ordered physiology. To achieve this, "clocks" throughout the body synchronize with 24-hour cycles in light,

Disclosures: None.
[a] Division of Human Genetics, Department of Pediatrics, Center for Chronobiology, Cincinnati Children's Hospital Medical Center, 240 Albert Sabin Way, Cincinnati, OH 45229, USA; [b] Division of Immunobiology, Department of Pediatrics, Center for Chronobiology, Cincinnati Children's Hospital Medical Center, 240 Albert Sabin Way, Cincinnati, OH 45229, USA; [c] Division of Pediatric Otolaryngology, Cincinnati Children's Hospital Medical Center, 3333 Burnet Avenue, Cincinnati, OH 45229, USA; [d] Division of Pulmonary and Sleep Medicine, Cincinnati Children's Hospital Medical Center, 3333 Burnet Avenue, Cincinnati, OH 45229, USA; [e] Department of Otolaryngology–Head and Neck Surgery, University of Cincinnati School of Medicine, 231 Albert Sabin Way, Cincinnati, OH 45267, USA
[1] Present address: 3333 Burnet Avenue, MLC 7008, Cincinnati, OH 45229.
* Corresponding author. 3333 Burnet Avenue, MLC 2018, Cincinnati, OH 45229.
E-mail address: David.Smith3@cchmc.org

Neurol Clin 37 (2019) 615–629
https://doi.org/10.1016/j.ncl.2019.03.004
0733-8619/19/© 2019 Elsevier Inc. All rights reserved.

neurologic.theclinics.com

activity, and other salient cues to enable appropriately aligned and adaptive biological functions.

The central clock in the suprachiasmatic nucleus (SCN) of the hypothalamus receives light input from the retina and transmits time-of-day cues to cellular clocks throughout the rest of the brain and body.[1] In this way, the SCN organizes sleep-wake timing and also many aspects of peripheral physiology. At the cellular level, the clock is a feedback loop involving transcriptional activators (BMAL1, CLOCK, NPAS2) and repressors (CRYs and PERs) that generates a 24-hour molecular oscillation and drives waves of expression in thousands of target genes. Half of mammalian protein-coding genes are rhythmically expressed somewhere in the body,[2,3] driving dozens of physiologic functions.[4]

In the brain, key steps in intercellular signaling are time-of-day regulated, from transmitter synthesis[5,6] to degradation[7,8] (**Fig. 1**A). Other fundamental neural processes, including endocytosis/exocytosis,[9] waste removal,[10,11] regulation of synaptic strength,[12–14] and permeability of the brain[15] and cerebrospinal fluid[16] to blood, also show daily variation. Therefore, it is not surprising that circadian disruption and neurologic disease often go hand in hand. Most neurodegenerative (eg, Alzheimer, Parkinson, Huntington) and psychiatric diseases (eg, schizophrenia, bipolar disorder,

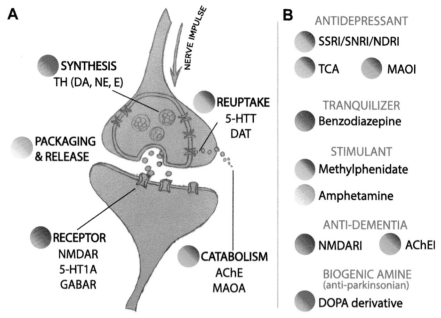

Fig. 1. Daily variation in mammalian neurotransmission. (A) Protein-level 24-hour variation at points in neurotransmitter life cycle: synthesis, packaging/release, reception, reuptake, and catabolism. (B) Standard medical therapies in neuropsychiatric or neurodegenerative disease. Those listed have primary targets whose abundance and/or function were shown to be time dependent somewhere in the mammalian brain (see **Table 1**). DOPA, dihydroxyphenylalanine; 5-HT, serotonin; 5-HTT, serotonin transporter; AChE, acetylcholinesterase; AChEI, acetylcholinesterase inhibitor; E, epinephrine; MAOA, monoamine oxidase A; MAOI, monoamine oxidase inhibitor; NDRI, norepinephrine and dopamine reuptake inhibitor; NE, norepinephrine; NMDAR, N-methyl-D-aspartate receptor; SNRI, selective serotonin and norepinephrine reuptake inhibitor; SSRI, selective serotonin reuptake inhibitor; TH, tyrosine hydroxylase.

and depression) are accompanied by sleep fragmentation and circadian rhythm disorders (SFCRDs) (as reviewed in Refs.[17–19]). Many of these diseases are without effective therapies, increasing in prevalence, and represent enormous unmet medical needs.

Circadian Disruption: Chicken or Egg?

Although the association between neurologic disease and SFCRD is well established,[20–22] the direction of causation remains uncertain. This association was a topic in prior reviews[17,23–25] and continues to pose a challenge in research and patient care.

There is genetic evidence that disruptions to the circadian system may be causal factors in the development of mental illness. Single nucleotide polymorphisms (SNPs) in several human circadian clock genes (CLOCK, BMAL1, NPAS2, PER2, CRY1, TEF, RORB) were associated with incidence and severity of attention-deficit/hyperactivity disorder (ADHD),[26,27] schizophrenia,[28,29] major depressive disorder (MDD),[30] bipolar disorder (BP),[31,32] posttraumatic stress disorder,[33] and seasonal-affective disorder.[34] All these diseases are complex, multigenic, and distinct from one another. It is noteworthy that so-called circadian entrainment was the top enriched pathway from the small set of 23 clinically relevant genes common to bipolar disorder (BP), schizophrenia, and autism.[35]

Studies of shift workers provide additional support for a causal link between circadian disruption and mental illnesses. Rotating schedules can lead to the loss of proper temporal coordination between organ systems (ie, circadian misalignment). These people have an increased risk of major depression and other mood disorders,[36,37] likely a consequence of chronic circadian misalignment.

Shift work is also associated with the risk of dementia,[38,39] suggesting that SFCRD may be a primary contributor in neurodegenerative disease as well. In Parkinson and Lewy body disease, rapid eye movement (REM) sleep disorders can manifest decades before the hallmark parkinsonian symptoms.[40] Early (presymptomatic) SFCRD is also seen in Alzheimer disease (AD) and other neurodegenerative disorders.[41,42] However, experiments in animals showed that early does not necessarily imply causal.[43,44] For example, in a mouse model of AD, the deposition of β-amyloid preceded the onset of sleep abnormalities, and its removal restored normal circadian rhythms.[44]

So, is SFCRD a primary contributor to neurodegenerative disease? It is difficult to say. Two studies linked SNPs in BMAL1 and CLOCK with incidence of AD,[45–47] but the associations were only significant in the subpopulation without the AD-risk allele apolipoprotein E (APOE e4). Although small, these studies suggest that the impact of genetic disruptions to the clock on dementia depends on genetic makeup, as expected in a multifactorial disease. Regardless of underlying cause, abnormal sleep-wake patterns can occur very early in neurodegenerative disease, predict risk of progression (in both animal[48–50] and clinical studies[51,52]), and are a major primary complaint from patients seen in neurology clinics.

Where Do Sleep and Circadian Medicine Fit in?

Sleep medicine is an interdisciplinary field based on the diagnosis and treatment of sleep disorders. Therapeutic modalities are broad and may or may not directly address circadian disruption (eg, cognitive behavior therapy for insomnia, medical therapy for symptoms of narcolepsy, or surgical therapy for resistant obstructive sleep apnea). In contrast, circadian medicine is intended to specifically incorporate knowledge of 24-hour biological rhythms to administer more effective treatment.

There are 2 broad approaches for circadian medicine. In the first, the therapeutic target is directly or indirectly the molecular oscillator (discussed later). Light therapy for phase disorders is the hallmark example and is effective at consolidating sleep in dementia.[53] In addition to light, drugs (eg, melatonin, zolpidem, tasimelteon) and diet[54] can also modulate the clock's amplitude or phase to potentially influence neurologic health.

A second approach in circadian medicine is intended to harmonize treatment with the clock's rhythmic outputs (discussed later). Timing the administration of a drug to coincide with peak levels of its physiologic target showed clinical benefits in hypertension, hypercholesterolemia, cancer, and several other areas.[55] Some of the key pathways targeted by standard-of-care drugs in neurology (monoamine and gamma-aminobutyric acid [GABA] neurotransmission, and others) are circadian regulated in the mammalian brain (**Fig. 1**). Can time of day be leveraged to improve existing treatments?

This article highlights how advances in circadian biology might translate to neurologic patient care. It focuses on neuropsychiatric and neurodegenerative conditions because they (1) share the common feature of SFCRD, and (2) are areas of high unmet medical need.

TREATING THE BRAIN'S CLOCK

Multiple factors lead to SFCRD in patients with dementia, including normal age-related changes, disease pathophysiology, medical comorbidities, side effects from medications, environmental and behavioral factors (eg, inadequate sleep hygiene), or some combination thereof.[56] Regardless of cause, sleep disorders impair cognition[57] and are a common cause of institutionalization in patients with dementia.[58] Consolidating sleep can markedly improve quality of life for the patients and caregivers.[59] However, clinicians face major challenges in achieving this.

Which Therapy in Which Patients, and When?

Options for treating sleep disruption include drug or light therapy, cognitive-behavioral intervention, and sleep hygiene recommendations. Although each of these affects the circadian clock, the mechanisms (and outcomes) are varied. Problematically, it is not clear which patients are the best candidates for a particular treatment. For example, sedative-hypnotics (ie, benzodiazepines) are widely used to treat sleep onset insomnia.[60] The Canadian Institute for Health reported 15% benzodiazepine use in the community, increasing to 30% in long-term care facilities[61] where half of the residents aged 80 years or older have dementia.[62] However, the American Academy of Sleep Medicine (AASM) strongly recommends against sleep-promoting medications to treat sleep-wake rhythm disorder in elderly demented patients[63] because of fall-related injuries[64] and impaired cognition.[65] This type of discordance between guidelines and practice is common in sleep medicine, and likely caused by reliance on therapies that are not well supported by large clinical trials and treatment practices that are driven by anecdotal experience.

The use of nonpharmacologic therapies for SFCRD in neurodegenerative disease is also equivocal. The AASM recommends bright light therapy (BLT) for patients with sleep and circadian rhythm disorders,[66,67] which can improve total sleep time in patients with dementia.[68] However, BLT was not effective for all SFCRD-related symptoms (eg, daytime behavior) in this patient population, and in some cases even exacerbated the symptoms.[69] How can the inconsistent results be explained?

One possibility is that clinicians have not fully delineated the appropriate timing of treatment. Guidelines for BLT recommend exposure before bedtime (to delay sleep phase) or on awakening (to advance sleep phase).[67] Critically, in order for BLT to impose strong and properly phased sleep-wake rhythms, it must be administered in narrow windows of circadian clock time, which presents a challenge. For example, in elderly patients with irregular sleep-wake patterns, it is difficult to measure circadian phase using current clinical tools, and therefore difficult to know when BLT is likely to be most effective. This difficulty is further complicated by the SCN becoming less responsive to light stimuli as people age,[70] emphasizing the importance of proper timing of administration in this population.

Are Some Therapies Worsening Sleep Fragmentation and Circadian Rhythm Disorders?

All of the major psychotherapeutic drug classes can affect sleep architecture (**Table 1**). For example, treatment-induced insomnia occurred in close to a quarter of patients taking venlafaxine for generalized anxiety disorders.[71] Although the mechanisms are broadly understood (eg, GABA agonists produce sedative effects), the specific effects on the central clock and sleep homeostat are not clear. This uncertainty is important when clinicians are trying to determine the primary and secondary causes of sleep disruption: will this patient require (1) therapy for a primary sleep disorder or (2) changes to medications prescribed for the neurologic disease? It is even more complex in patients that require polydrug therapy.

There is an even broader challenge here: because of the inextricable link between sleep, circadian rhythms, and neural function, it is not always clear what is being treated. Indeed, recent studies suggest that the benefits from some psychotherapeutics (eg, lithium, selective serotonin reuptake inhibitors [SSRIs]) may derive from their effects on the circadian system.[72] The SSRI citalopram, prescribed for depression and anxiety, acutely increased the sensitivity of the human circadian system to light,[73] which may realign the circadian clock and contribute to the drug's antidepressant effect.

Moving Sleep and Circadian Medicine Forward

Advancements in sleep medicine will depend on improved approaches to (1) measure internal circadian phase, (2) reliably shift circadian phase, (3) strengthen rhythms (ie, amplitude), and (4) understand how SFCRD fits in the context of other diseases (eg, neurodegeneration).

Table 1
Effects of common psychotherapeutic drug classes on sleep

Drug Class	Time to Sleep Onset	Sleep Continuity	Slow Wave Sleep	REM Sleep
SSRI	Increased	Decreased	Decreased	Decreased
SNRI	Unchanged	Decreased	Decreased	Decreased
MAOI	Increased	Decreased	Unchanged	Decreased
TCA	Decreased	Increased	Unchanged	Decreased
Trazodone	Decreased	Increased	Increased	Decreased
Antipsychotic	Decreased	Increased	Increased	Decreased
Anxiolytic	Decreased	Increased	Decreased	Decreased

These are general class effects on sleep. Each drug has its own profile.

Abbreviations: MAOI, monoamine oxidase inhibitor; SNRI, serotonin norepinephrine reuptake inhibitor; SSRI, selective serotonin reuptake inhibitor; TCA, tricyclic antidepressant.

Adapted from Barkoukis TJ, Avidan AY, service) S (online. Review of Sleep Medicine; with permission.

Current methods for determining internal circadian phase are limited and not used clinically. The gold-standard dim-light melatonin onset (DLMO) assay is based on the circadian clock–regulated evening increase in melatonin levels[74] and requires the serial sampling of saliva over a 24-hour period. DLMO is time consuming, costly, difficult to standardize, and therefore rarely used to diagnose circadian rhythm disorders. However, last year 3 separate studies showed the feasibility of gene expression signatures from 1 or 2 minimally invasive (skin or blood) samples to determine a person's circadian phase.[75–77] As mentioned, the efficacy of BLT, and potentially all therapies aimed at circadian realignment, depends on the time at which they are administered. A single-sample point-of-use biomarker could therefore have broad diagnostic and therapeutic value.

In addition to light, exercise and feeding can influence the circadian clock. Although not routinely used in practice, exercise can help consolidate sleep in the elderly.[78,79] The type and timing of nutrient intake can also influence circadian clocks in health.[49,80] In order to determine the use for these newer methods to treat SFCRD, larger clinical trials must be completed. New methods for determining circadian time should lead to guidelines for how and when these therapies should be given.

Circadian disruption occurs presymptomatically in AD,[41] as mentioned. Several genes implicated in neurodegenerative (and neuropsychiatric) disease are circadian regulated in mice,[2] including AD-risk genes β-secretase enzyme 1 (Bace1), Bace2, and APOE in the hippocampus.[81] There is evidence that genetically disrupted clock function can predispose to neurodegeneration.[45,47,82] Can treatment of SFCRD, if early and effective, attenuate or delay AD?

LEVERAGING THE CLOCK'S RHYTHMIC OUTPUT
Timing Treatment to Target Dynamics

Timing treatment to coincide with daily rhythms in clock output is not new. The short-acting statin, simvastatin, is more effective at reducing lipid levels if taken at night, when its target, the rate-limiting enzyme in cholesterol biosynthesis, is at its peak levels.[83] However, apart from simvastatin, which has US Food and Drug Administration–labeled time-of-day dosing instructions, circadian time has had very little role in drug development or clinical practice. One reason for this is a lack of understanding about how the circadian clock regulates human physiology and pathophysiology.

However, a series of advances have renewed translational interest. First, circadian regulation is far more pervasive than previously appreciated.[2,4] In a multitissue time-series study in mice, nearly half of the protein-coding genome was circadian regulated somewhere in the body. In the nervous system alone, many basic neural functions have been shown to vary by time of day, as mentioned earlier. Second, genome-wide and systems-wide circadian profiling, historically limited to time-series studies in animal models, is now feasible in humans. A recent study by our group applied a bioinformatic approach called cyclic ordering by periodic structure (CYCLOPS)[84] to assemble a population-scale atlas of circadian gene expression across 13 different human tissue types.[3] The study found ~1000 genes that were rhythmically expressed somewhere in the human body that encode known drug targets.

Are there neurologic therapies whose efficacy or safety might depend on time of dosing?

Time for Targeting Neurotransmission

Monoamine neurotransmission is a major therapeutic target in neurology. Six different serotonin-specific and norepinephrine-specific reuptake inhibitor drugs(indicated for depression, anxiety, and other mood disorders) are among the top 50 most prescribed drugs in the United States.[85] The first SSRI (fluoxetine/Prozac) was developed in the 1970s[86] based on evidence of low serotonin and/or norepinephrine levels in depression.[87] However, although widely prescribed, many patients (most, by some accounts) do not benefit from SSRI therapy.[88]

Accumulating evidence has shown that monoamine transmitters are circadian regulated in brain loci implicated in arousal and mood, as reviewed by Albrecht[89] (**Fig. 1**B; **Table 2**). However, knowledge of these 24-hour dynamics has not factored into clinical practice or drug development. Most SSRI/serotonin norepinephrine reuptake inhibitor formulations are long acting (half-lives >12 hours). Could a short-acting SSRI be used to restore normal 24-hour rhythms in synaptic serotonin? In a mouse model of moodlike behavior, effects of the short-acting SSRI milnacipran were circadian-time dependent.[90] Future studies should test whether these findings are generalizable. Several other drug classes routinely prescribed in neuropsychiatric and neurodegenerative disease also target time-dependent physiology (see **Fig. 1**B, **Table 2**).

Table 2
Drug classes with time-dependent targets in mammalian brain tissues

Drug Class	Approved Uses	Time-dependent Target (Protein Levels or Function)	Study
SSRI/SNRI	MDD, GAD, SAD, PD, OCD, PMDD, PTSD, bulimia nervosa	5-HTT	Cortex (human)[103]
NDRI	MDD	DAT	Striatum (mouse)[104]
Methylphenidate	ADD, narcolepsy	DAT	Striatum (mouse)[104]
Amphetamine	ADD, narcolepsy	Vesicle recycling machinery	SCN (mouse)[9]
MAOI	MDD, atypical depression, BP, AD, PD	MAOA	VTA, striatum (mouse)[7]
AChEI	AD, LBD, PD, MG, SCZ	AChE	Cerebrum, cerebellum, medulla, optic lobe (rat)[8]
NMDAR antagonist	AD, PD, drug-induced extrapyramidal reactions	NMDARs	SCN, motor cortex (rat)[105,106]
Benzodiazepine	Insomnia, GAD, PD	GABA$_A$ receptors	Cerebral cortex, SCN (hamster)[107,108]
Biogenic amine	PD	TH	VTA, nucleus accumbens, pineal gland (rat)[109,110]

References are not exhaustive, and many other known targets of these drugs in neuropsychiatric and neurodegenerative disease were shown to be circadian regulated at the transcriptional level but are not shown here.

Abbreviations: AChE, acetylcholinesterase; AChEI, acetylcholinesterase inhibitor; ADD, attention-deficit disorders; BP, bipolar disorder; DAT, dopamine transporter; GAD, generalized anxiety disorder; 5-HTT, serotonin transporter; LBD, Lewy body dementias; MAOA, monoamine oxidase A; MG, myasthenia gravis; NDRI, norepinephrine and dopamine reuptake inhibitor; NMDAR, N-methyl-D-aspartate receptor; OCD, obsessive-compulsive disorder; PD, panic disorder; PMDD, premenstrual dysphoric disorder; PTSD, posttraumatic stress disorder; SAD, social anxiety disorder; SCZ, schizophrenia; TH, tyrosine hydroxylase; VTA, ventral tegmental area.

Timing Off Targets and Drug Disposition

Alternatively, drug delivery can be timed to coincide with trough levels of an undesired target. The idea here is that adverse drug-related events can be minimized if drug exposure is out of phase with the mechanisms responsible for the adverse events. A study of the influence of dosing time on the effects of the antipsychotic aripiprazole (ARPZ) provides (retrospective) clinical support for this strategy.[91] ARPZ can cause metabolic abnormalities because of off-target antagonism of D2 dopamine receptors (D2Rs) in the pancreas. This antagonism can lead to weight gain, a primary reason for drug discontinuation. The study found that patients who took ARPZ at bedtime had worse metabolic outcomes (poor lipid profiles) compared with morning dosing.[91] The precise mechanism needs to be verified, but it was proposed that pancreatic D2R levels are clock regulated, highest at bedtime, and thus antagonism at this time leads to abnormally increased insulin levels during sleep and consequent metabolic dysregulation.

Another approach is to harmonize the administration of a drug with rhythms in its disposition. Passage through the blood-brain barrier (BBB) is a challenge in drug development; increased doses can deliver more drug to the central nervous system (CNS), but toxicity in the periphery can be dose limiting. Recent work in *Drosophila* showed a clinically relevant time dependency in BBB permeability,[92] and evidence suggests a similar mechanism may exist in mammals.[15] Time-dependent BBB permeability could be leveraged to improve therapeutic windows for both CNS-targeting and peripheral nervous system (PNS)–targeting drugs. As an example of the latter, there is a need in peripheral neuropathic pain for drugs with better-tolerated CNS-side-effect profiles.[93,94] Future models will define the scope of potential benefit from harmonizing treatment with BBB permeability.

Very few clinical trials have tested the influence of time of day on CNS-targeting and PNS-targeting agents.[95–98] As the understanding of circadian-expressed targets and physiology in neurologic disease expands, so does the potential for time-stipulated therapy.

CONCLUDING THOUGHTS
The next Decade: Implementing Circadian Medicine

There are unmet needs for more effective therapies in several areas of neurology. Drug development in neurodegenerative disease is marked with pivotal failures,[99] and controversy surrounds the clinical value of standard-of-care therapies in mental illness.[100] In 2018, soon after unsuccessful attempts to translate molecular targets into efficacious new therapies, Pfizer, the world's third largest pharmaceutical company, announced plans to abandon all research and development into new neuroscience programs.[101]

Circadian medicine alone is not a panacea. However, recent advances in the understanding of 24-hour dynamics in physiology and disease create a path for near-term improvements in medicine. This article concludes with 3 specific clinical scenarios of how technologic advances in circadian biology might change patient care in the next decade.

1. By administering a single minimally invasive test for internal time, a clinician diagnoses circadian sleep-wake phase disorders in patients. Biomarkers of internal time based on gene expression signatures can replace DLMO, actigraphy, and unreliable sleep diaries.
2. The neurologist stipulates timing of light therapy, exercise, and feeding to strengthen clock function in a patient with low-amplitude or irregular sleep-wake rhythms, such as in neurodegenerative disorders. The circadian clock in the SCN

is maximally sensitive to light-resetting during narrow windows of time (phases). With an accurate test for internal phase, treatment can be delivered at the most appropriate time.

3. Guided by a map of 24-hour dynamics in 5-HT neurotransmission in the brain, researchers initiate a clinical trial to test administration-time dependency of SSRIs in depression. Current maps of circadian dynamics in the human brain remain poorly resolved, but this is likely to change. Genomic repositories are ever growing, some with extensive coverage across brain regions (eg, GTEx[102]). A circadian human brain atlas is foreseeable, and should spark mechanism-based prospective trials in circadian medicine.

REFERENCES

1. Weaver DR. Introduction to circadian rhythms and mechanisms of circadian oscillations. In: Gumz ML, editor. Circadian clocks: role in health and disease. New York: Springer New York; 2016. p. 1–55.
2. Zhang R, Lahens NF, Ballance HI, et al. A circadian gene expression atlas in mammals: implications for biology and medicine. Proc Natl Acad Sci U S A 2014;111(45):16219–24.
3. Ruben MD, Wu G, Smith DF, et al. A database of tissue-specific rhythmically expressed human genes has potential applications in circadian medicine. Sci Transl Med 2018;10(458). https://doi.org/10.1126/scitranslmed.aat8806.
4. Skarke C, Lahens NF, Rhoades SD, et al. A pilot characterization of the human chronobiome. Sci Rep 2017;7(1):17141.
5. Yu X, Zecharia A, Zhang Z, et al. Circadian factor BMAL1 in histaminergic neurons regulates sleep architecture. Curr Biol 2014;24(23):2838–44.
6. Chung S, Lee EJ, Yun S, et al. Impact of circadian nuclear receptor REV-ERBα on midbrain dopamine production and mood regulation. Cell 2014;157(4): 858–68.
7. Hampp G, Ripperger JA, Houben T, et al. Regulation of monoamine oxidase A by circadian-clock components implies clock influence on mood. Curr Biol 2008;18(9):678–83.
8. Mohan C, Radha E. Circadian rhythm in acetylcholinesterase activity during aging of the central nervous system. Life Sci 1974;15(2):231–7.
9. Deery MJ, Maywood ES, Chesham JE, et al. Proteomic analysis reveals the role of synaptic vesicle cycling in sustaining the suprachiasmatic circadian clock. Curr Biol 2009;19(23):2031–6.
10. Xie L, Kang H, Xu Q, et al. Sleep drives metabolite clearance from the adult brain. Science 2013;342(6156):373–7.
11. Lundgaard I, Lu ML, Yang E, et al. Glymphatic clearance controls state-dependent changes in brain lactate concentration. J Cereb Blood Flow Metab 2017;37(6):2112–24.
12. Tononi G, Cirelli C. Sleep and the price of plasticity: from synaptic and cellular homeostasis to memory consolidation and integration. Neuron 2014;81(1): 12–34.
13. Vyazovskiy VV, Cirelli C, Pfister-Genskow M, et al. Molecular and electrophysiological evidence for net synaptic potentiation in wake and depression in sleep. Nat Neurosci 2008;11(2):200–8.
14. Hinard V, Mikhail C, Pradervand S, et al. Key electrophysiological, molecular, and metabolic signatures of sleep and wakefulness revealed in primary cortical cultures. J Neurosci 2012;32(36):12506–17.

15. Kervezee L, Hartman R, van den Berg D-J, et al. Diurnal variation in P-glycoprotein-mediated transport and cerebrospinal fluid turnover in the brain. AAPS J 2014;16(5):1029–37.

16. Pan W, Cornélissen G, Halberg F, et al. Selected contribution: circadian rhythm of tumor necrosis factor-alpha uptake into mouse spinal cord. J Appl Physiol 2002;92(3):1357–62 [discussion: 1356].

17. Vadnie CA, McClung CA. Circadian Rhythm Disturbances in Mood Disorders: Insights into the Role of the Suprachiasmatic Nucleus. Neural Plast 2017; 2017:1504507.

18. Videnovic A, Lazar AS, Barker RA, et al. "The clocks that time us"–circadian rhythms in neurodegenerative disorders. Nat Rev Neurol 2014;10(12):683–93.

19. Iranzo A. Sleep in neurodegenerative diseases. Sleep Med Clin 2016;11(1): 1–18.

20. Harper DG, Volicer L, Stopa EG, et al. Disturbance of endogenous circadian rhythm in aging and Alzheimer disease. Am J Geriatr Psychiatry 2005;13(5): 359–68.

21. Hatfield CF, Herbert J, van Someren EJW, et al. Disrupted daily activity/rest cycles in relation to daily cortisol rhythms of home-dwelling patients with early Alzheimer's dementia. Brain 2004;127(Pt 5):1061–74.

22. Bliwise DL, Mercaldo ND, Avidan AY, et al. Sleep disturbance in dementia with Lewy bodies and Alzheimer's disease: a multicenter analysis. Dement Geriatr Cogn Disord 2011;31(3):239–46.

23. Hastings MH, Goedert M. Circadian clocks and neurodegenerative diseases: time to aggregate? Curr Opin Neurobiol 2013;23(5):880–7.

24. Phan T, Malkani R. Sleep and circadian rhythm disruption and stress intersect in Alzheimer's disease. Neurobiol Stress 2018. https://doi.org/10.1016/j.ynstr.2018. 10.001.

25. Musiek ES, Holtzman DM. Mechanisms linking circadian clocks, sleep, and neurodegeneration. Science 2016;354(6315):1004–8.

26. Kissling C, Retz W, Wiemann S, et al. A polymorphism at the 3'-untranslated region of the CLOCK gene is associated with adult attention-deficit hyperactivity disorder. Am J Med Genet B Neuropsychiatr Genet 2008;147(3):333–8.

27. Xu X, Breen G, Chen C-K, et al. Association study between a polymorphism at the 3'-untranslated region of CLOCK gene and attention deficit hyperactivity disorder. Behav Brain Funct 2010;6:48.

28. Takao T, Tachikawa H, Kawanishi Y, et al. CLOCK gene T3111C polymorphism is associated with Japanese schizophrenics: a preliminary study. Eur Neuropsychopharmacol 2007;17(4):273–6.

29. Kishi T, Kitajima T, Ikeda M, et al. Association study of clock gene (CLOCK) and schizophrenia and mood disorders in the Japanese population. Eur Arch Psychiatry Clin Neurosci 2009;259(5):293–7.

30. Benedetti F, Radaelli D, Bernasconi A, et al. Clock genes beyond the clock: CLOCK genotype biases neural correlates of moral valence decision in depressed patients. Genes Brain Behav 2008;7(1):20–5.

31. Serretti A, Benedetti F, Mandelli L, et al. Genetic dissection of psychopathological symptoms: insomnia in mood disorders and CLOCK gene polymorphism. Am J Med Genet B Neuropsychiatr Genet 2003;121B(1):35–8.

32. Soria V, Martínez-Amorós E, Escaramís G, et al. Differential association of circadian genes with mood disorders: CRY1 and NPAS2 are associated with unipolar major depression and CLOCK and VIP with bipolar disorder. Neuropsychopharmacology 2010;35(6):1279–89.

33. Linnstaedt SD, Pan Y, Mauck MC, et al. Evaluation of the association between genetic variants in circadian rhythm genes and posttraumatic stress symptoms identifies a potential functional allele in the transcription factor TEF. Front Psychiatry 2018;9:597.
34. Partonen T, Treutlein J, Alpman A, et al. Three circadian clock genes Per2, Arntl, and Npas2 contribute to winter depression. Ann Med 2007;39(3):229–38.
35. Khanzada NS, Butler MG, Manzardo AM. geneanalytics pathway analysis and genetic overlap among autism spectrum disorder, bipolar disorder and schizophrenia. Int J Mol Sci 2017;18(3). https://doi.org/10.3390/ijms18030527.
36. Asaoka S, Aritake S, Komada Y, et al. Factors associated with shift work disorder in nurses working with rapid-rotation schedules in Japan: the nurses' sleep health project. Chronobiol Int 2013;30(4):628–36.
37. Scott AJ, Monk TH, Brink LL. Shiftwork as a risk factor for depression: a pilot study. Int J Occup Environ Health 1997;3(Supplement 2):S2–9.
38. Bokenberger K, Sjölander A, Dahl Aslan AK, et al. Shift work and risk of incident dementia: a study of two population-based cohorts. Eur J Epidemiol 2018; 33(10):977–87.
39. Jørgensen JT, Karlsen S, Stayner L, et al. Shift work and overall and cause-specific mortality in the Danish nurse cohort. Scand J Work Environ Health 2017;43(2):117–26.
40. Boeve BF. Idiopathic REM sleep behaviour disorder in the development of Parkinson's disease. Lancet Neurol 2013;12(5):469–82.
41. Musiek ES, Bhimasani M, Zangrilli MA, et al. Circadian rest-activity pattern changes in aging and preclinical Alzheimer disease. JAMA Neurol 2018; 75(5):582–90.
42. Abbott SM, Videnovic A. Chronic sleep disturbance and neural injury: links to neurodegenerative disease. Nat Sci Sleep 2016;8:55–61.
43. Pallier PN, Maywood ES, Zheng Z, et al. Pharmacological imposition of sleep slows cognitive decline and reverses dysregulation of circadian gene expression in a transgenic mouse model of Huntington's disease. J Neurosci 2007; 27(29):7869–78.
44. Roh JH, Huang Y, Bero AW, et al. Disruption of the sleep-wake cycle and diurnal fluctuation of β-amyloid in mice with Alzheimer's disease pathology. Sci Transl Med 2012;4(150):150ra122.
45. Chen Q, Peng XD, Huang CQ, et al. Association between ARNTL (BMAL1) rs2278749 polymorphism T >C and susceptibility to Alzheimer disease in a Chinese population. Genet Mol Res 2015;14(4):18515–22.
46. Chen H-F, Huang C-Q, You C, et al. Polymorphism of CLOCK gene rs 4580704 C> G is associated with susceptibility of Alzheimer's disease in a Chinese population. Arch Med Res 2013;44(3):203–7.
47. Yang Y-K, Peng X-D, Li Y-H, et al. The polymorphism of CLOCK gene 3111T/C C>T is associated with susceptibility of Alzheimer disease in Chinese population. J Investig Med 2013;61(7):1084–7.
48. Zhu Y, Zhan G, Fenik P, et al. Chronic sleep disruption advances the temporal progression of tauopathy in P301S mutant mice. J Neurosci 2018. https://doi.org/10.1523/JNEUROSCI.0275-18.2018.
49. Whittaker DS, Loh DH, Wang H-B, et al. Circadian-based treatment strategy effective in the BACHD mouse model of Huntington's disease. J Biol Rhythms 2018;33(5):535–54.
50. Kang J-E, Lim MM, Bateman RJ, et al. Amyloid-beta dynamics are regulated by orexin and the sleep-wake cycle. Science 2009;326(5955):1005–7.

51. Lim ASP, Kowgier M, Yu L, et al. Sleep fragmentation and the risk of incident Alzheimer's disease and cognitive decline in older persons. Sleep 2013;36(7): 1027–32.

52. Benedict C, Byberg L, Cedernaes J, et al. Self-reported sleep disturbance is associated with Alzheimer's disease risk in men. Alzheimers Dement 2015; 11(9):1090–7.

53. Hanford N, Figueiro M. Light therapy and Alzheimer's disease and related dementia: past, present, and future. J Alzheimers Dis 2013;33(4):913–22.

54. Wehrens SMT, Christou S, Isherwood C, et al. Meal timing regulates the human circadian system. Curr Biol 2017;27(12):1768–75.e3.

55. Kaur G, Phillips CL, Wong K, et al. Timing of administration: for commonly-prescribed medicines in Australia. Pharmaceutics 2016;8(2). https://doi.org/10.3390/pharmaceutics8020013.

56. McCurry SM, Reynolds CF, Ancoli-Israel S, et al. Treatment of sleep disturbance in Alzheimer's disease. Sleep Med Rev 2000;4(6):603–28.

57. Vitiello MV, Borson S. Sleep disturbances in patients with Alzheimer's disease. CNS Drugs 2001;15(10):777–96.

58. Hope T, Keene J, Gedling K, et al. Predictors of institutionalization for people with dementia living at home with a carer. Int J Geriatr Psychiatry 1998;13(10): 682–90.

59. Deschenes CL, McCurry SM. Current treatments for sleep disturbances in individuals with dementia. Curr Psychiatry Rep 2009;11(1):20–6.

60. McCall WV. Diagnosis and management of insomnia in older people. J Am Geriatr Soc 2005;53(7 Suppl):S272–7.

61. Proulx J, Hunt J. Drug use among seniors on public drug programs in Canada, 2012. Healthc Q 2015;18(1):11–3.

62. Wong SL, Gilmour H, Ramage-Morin PL. Alzheimer's disease and other dementias in Canada. Health Rep 2016;27(5):11–6.

63. Auger RR, Burgess HJ, Emens JS, et al. Clinical practice guideline for the treatment of intrinsic circadian rhythm sleep-wake disorders: advanced sleep-wake phase disorder (ASWPD), delayed sleep-wake phase disorder (DSWPD), non-24-hour sleep-wake rhythm disorder (N24SWD), and irregular sleep-wake rhythm disorder (ISWRD). An update for 2015. J Clin Sleep Med 2015;11(10): 1199–236.

64. Tamblyn R, Abrahamowicz M, du Berger R, et al. A 5-year prospective assessment of the risk associated with individual benzodiazepines and doses in new elderly users. J Am Geriatr Soc 2005;53(2):233–41.

65. By the American Geriatrics Society 2015 Beers Criteria Update Expert Panel. American Geriatrics Society 2015 updated beers criteria for potentially inappropriate medication use in older adults. J Am Geriatr Soc 2015;63(11):2227–46.

66. Chesson AL, Littner M, Davila D, et al. Practice parameters for the use of light therapy in the treatment of sleep disorders. Sleep 1999;22(5):641–60.

67. Morgenthaler TI, Lee-Chiong T, Alessi C, et al. Practice parameters for the clinical evaluation and treatment of circadian rhythm sleep disorders. Sleep 2007; 30(11):1445–59.

68. Lyketsos CG, Lindell Veiel L, Baker A, et al. A randomized, controlled trial of bright light therapy for agitated behaviors in dementia patients residing in long-term care. Int J Geriatr Psychiatry 1999;14(7):520–5.

69. Barrick AL, Sloane PD, Williams CS, et al. Impact of ambient bright light on agitation in dementia. Int J Geriatr Psychiatry 2010;25(10):1013–21.

70. Skene DJ, Swaab DF. Melatonin rhythmicity: effect of age and Alzheimer's disease. Exp Gerontol 2003;38(1–2):199–206.
71. Wichniak A, Wierzbicka A, Walęcka M, et al. Effects of Antidepressants on Sleep. Curr Psychiatry Rep 2017;19(9):63.
72. Rybakowski JK, Dmitrzak-Weglar M, Kliwicki S, et al. Polymorphism of circadian clock genes and prophylactic lithium response. Bipolar Disord 2014;16(2):151–8.
73. McGlashan EM, Nandam LS, Vidafar P, et al. The SSRI citalopram increases the sensitivity of the human circadian system to light in an acute dose. Psychopharmacology 2018. https://doi.org/10.1007/s00213-018-5019-0.
74. Lewy AJ, Cutler NL, Sack RL. The endogenous melatonin profile as a marker for circadian phase position. J Biol Rhythms 1999;14(3):227–36.
75. Wu G, Ruben MD, Schmidt RE, et al. Population level rhythms in human skin: implications for circadian medicine. bioRxiv 2018. https://doi.org/10.1101/301820.
76. Wittenbrink N, Ananthasubramaniam B, Münch M, et al. High-accuracy determination of internal circadian time from a single blood sample. J Clin Invest 2018. https://doi.org/10.1172/JCI120874.
77. Braun R, Kath WL, Iwanaszko M, et al. Universal method for robust detection of circadian state from gene expression. Proc Natl Acad Sci U S A 2018. https://doi.org/10.1073/pnas.1800314115.
78. Baehr EK, Eastman CI, Revelle W, et al. Circadian phase-shifting effects of nocturnal exercise in older compared with young adults. Am J Physiol Regul Integr Comp Physiol 2003;284(6):R1542–50.
79. King AC, Oman RF, Brassington GS, et al. Moderate-intensity exercise and self-rated quality of sleep in older adults. A randomized controlled trial. JAMA 1997;277(1):32–7.
80. Oike H. Modulation of circadian clocks by nutrients and food factors. Biosci Biotechnol Biochem 2017;81(5):863–70.
81. Ma Z, Jiang W, Zhang EE. Orexin signaling regulates both the hippocampal clock and the circadian oscillation of Alzheimer's disease-risk genes. Sci Rep 2016;6:36035.
82. Gu Z, Wang B, Zhang Y-B, et al. Association of ARNTL and PER1 genes with Parkinson's disease: a case-control study of Han Chinese. Sci Rep 2015;5:15891.
83. Saito Y, Yoshida S, Nakaya N, et al. Comparison between morning and evening doses of simvastatin in hyperlipidemic subjects. A double-blind comparative study. Arterioscler Thromb 1991;11(4):816–26.
84. Anafi RC, Francey LJ, Hogenesch JB, et al. CYCLOPS reveals human transcriptional rhythms in health and disease. Proc Natl Acad Sci U S A 2017;114(20):5312–7.
85. Top 200 Prescribed Medicines of 2018. ClinCalc. 2018. Available at: http://clincalc.com/DrugStats/Top200Drugs.aspx. Accessed September 2018.
86. Wong DT, Horng JS, Bymaster FP, et al. A selective inhibitor of serotonin uptake: Lilly 110140, 3-(p-trifluoromethylphenoxy)-N-methyl-3-phenylpropylamine. Life Sci 1974;15(3):471–9.
87. Schildkraut JJ. Neuropharmacology of the affective disorders. Annu Rev Pharmacol 1973;13:427–54.
88. Rush AJ, Trivedi MH, Wisniewski SR, et al. Acute and longer-term outcomes in depressed outpatients requiring one or several treatment steps: a STAR*D report. Am J Psychiatry 2006;163(11):1905–17.

89. Albrecht U. Molecular Mechanisms in Mood Regulation Involving the Circadian Clock. Front Neurol 2017;8:30.

90. Kawai H, Machida M, Ishibashi T, et al. Chronopharmacological Analysis of Antidepressant Activity of a Dual-Action Serotonin Noradrenaline Reuptake Inhibitor (SNRI), Milnacipran, in Rats. Biol Pharm Bull 2018;41(2):213–9.

91. Chipchura DA, Freyberg Z, Edwards C, et al. Does the time of drug administration alter the metabolic risk of aripiprazole? Front Psychiatry 2018;9:494.

92. Zhang SL, Yue Z, Arnold DM, et al. A circadian clock in the blood-brain barrier regulates xenobiotic efflux. Cell 2018;173(1):130–9.e10.

93. Murphy KL, Bethea JR, Fischer R. Neuropathic pain in multiple sclerosis—current therapeutic intervention and future treatment perspectives. In: Zagon IS, McLaughlin PJ, editors. Multiple sclerosis: perspectives in treatment and pathogenesis. Brisbane (AU): Codon Publications; 2017.

94. Finnerup NB, Attal N, Haroutounian S, et al. Pharmacotherapy for neuropathic pain in adults: a systematic review and meta-analysis. Lancet Neurol 2015; 14(2):162–73.

95. Badiyan SN, Ferraro DJ, Yaddanapudi S, et al. Impact of time of day on outcomes after stereotactic radiosurgery for non-small cell lung cancer brain metastases. Cancer 2013;119(19):3563–9.

96. Rahn DA 3rd, Ray DK, Schlesinger DJ, et al. Gamma knife radiosurgery for brain metastasis of nonsmall cell lung cancer: is there a difference in outcome between morning and afternoon treatment? Cancer 2011;117(2):414–20.

97. Chan S, Rowbottom L, McDonald R, et al. Could time of whole brain radiotherapy delivery impact overall survival in patients with multiple brain metastases? Ann Palliat Med 2016;5(4):267–79.

98. Shappell SA, Kearns GL, Valentine JL, et al. Chronopharmacokinetics and chronopharmacodynamics of dextromethamphetamine in man. J Clin Pharmacol 1996;36(11):1051–63.

99. Salloway S, Sperling R, Fox NC, et al. Two phase 3 trials of bapineuzumab in mild-to-moderate Alzheimer's disease. N Engl J Med 2014;370(4):322–33.

100. Kirsch I, Deacon BJ, Huedo-Medina TB, et al. Initial severity and antidepressant benefits: a meta-analysis of data submitted to the Food and Drug Administration. PLoS Med 2008;5(2):e45.

101. Terry M. Pfizer to cut 300 jobs as it ends Alzheimer's, Parkinson's quest | BioSpace. BioSpace; 2018. Available at: https://www.biospace.com/article/unique-pfizer-to-cut-300-jobs-as-it-ends-alzheimer-s-parkinson-s-quest/. Accessed October 23, 2018.

102. GTEx Consortium. The Genotype-Tissue Expression (GTEx) project. Nat Genet 2013;45(6):580–5.

103. Matheson GJ, Schain M, Almeida R, et al. Diurnal and seasonal variation of the brain serotonin system in healthy male subjects. Neuroimage 2015;112:225–31.

104. Ferris MJ, España RA, Locke JL, et al. Dopamine transporters govern diurnal variation in extracellular dopamine tone. Proc Natl Acad Sci U S A 2014; 111(26):E2751–9.

105. Bendová Z, Sumová A, Mikkelsen JD. Circadian and developmental regulation of N-methyl-d-aspartate-receptor 1 mRNA splice variants and N-methyl-d-aspartate-receptor 3 subunit expression within the rat suprachiasmatic nucleus. Neuroscience 2009;159(2):599–609.

106. Estrada-Rojo F, Morales-Gomez J, Coballase-Urrutia E, et al. Diurnal variation of NMDA receptor expression in the rat cerebral cortex is associated with traumatic brain injury damage. BMC Res Notes 2018;11(1):150.

107. Kanterewicz BI, Rosenstein RE, Golombek DA, et al. Daily variations in GABA receptor function in Syrian hamster cerebral cortex. Neurosci Lett 1995; 200(3):211–3.
108. Walton JC, McNeill JK 4th, Oliver KA, et al. Temporal regulation of GABAA receptor subunit expression: role in synaptic and extrasynaptic communication in the suprachiasmatic nucleus. eNeuro 2017;4(2). https://doi.org/10.1523/ENEURO.0352-16.2017.
109. McGeer EG, McGeer PL. Circadian rhythm in pineal tyrosine hydroxylase. Science 1966;153(3731):73–4.
110. Webb IC, Baltazar RM, Wang X, et al. Diurnal variations in natural and drug reward, mesolimbic tyrosine hydroxylase, and clock gene expression in the male rat. J Biol Rhythms 2009;24(6):465–76.

Moving?

Make sure your subscription moves with you!

To notify us of your new address, find your **Clinics Account Number** (located on your mailing label above your name), and contact customer service at:

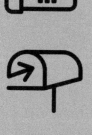

Email: journalscustomerservice-usa@elsevier.com

800-654-2452 (subscribers in the U.S. & Canada)
314-447-8871 (subscribers outside of the U.S. & Canada)

Fax number: 314-447-8029

Elsevier Health Sciences Division
Subscription Customer Service
3251 Riverport Lane
Maryland Heights, MO 63043

*To ensure uninterrupted delivery of your subscription, please notify us at least 4 weeks in advance of move.

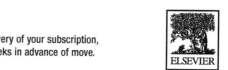

Printed and bound by CPI Group (UK) Ltd, Croydon, CR0 4YY

03/10/2024

01040407-0011